PILATES
BASICS

PILATES
BASICS

Master Pilates Fundamentals as You Balance,
Strengthen, and Align from Within

JILLIAN HESSEL

RODALE

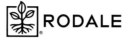

WE **INSPIRE** AND **ENABLE** PEOPLE TO IMPROVE
THEIR LIVES AND THE WORLD AROUND THEM

Printed in the United States of America on acid-free ∞, recycled ♻ paper

Editor: Christine Bucks

Cover and Interior Book Designer: Joanna Williams

Interior Illustrator: Nicole Kauffman

Cover Photographer: Ron Derhacopian

Interior Photographers: Adam Brown (pages 24, 48, 92, 136, 156); Ron Derhacopian (all except as noted); Ric Kokotovich (page 14)

Layout Designer: Donna Bellis

Copy Editors: Erana Bumbardatore, Diana R. Cobb

Product Specialist: Brenda Miller

Indexer: Nanette Bendyna

Rodale Organic Living Books

Executive Editor: Margot Schupf

Art Director: Patricia Field

Content Assembly Manager: Robert V. Anderson Jr.

Copy Manager: Nancy N. Bailey

Editorial Assistant: Sara Sellar

We're always happy to hear from you. For questions or comments concerning the editorial content of this book, please write to:

Rodale Book Readers' Service

33 East Minor Street

Emmaus, PA 18098

Look for other Rodale books wherever books are sold. Or call us at (800) 848-4735.

For more information about Rodale Organic Living magazines and books, visit us at:

www.rodale.com

Library of Congress Cataloging-in-Publication Data

Hessel, Jillian.
    Pilates basics : master pilates fundamentals as you strengthen, align, and balance from within / Jillian Hessel.
        p.   cm.
    Includes index.
    ISBN 0–87596–913–5 (pbk. : alk. paper)
    1. Pilates method.   I. Title.
RA781.H474   2003
613.7′1—dc21   2003002341

Distributed in the book trade by St. Martin's Press

2 4 6 8 10 9 7 5 3 1 paperback

CONTENTS

FOREWORD

Pearl Lang, former principal dancer of the Martha Graham Company, was the one who suggested I see Joseph Pilates—then largely unknown—to help me resume dancing after two major knee operations. This was back in 1954. Little did I know how much of an impact Joseph Pilates (along with his wife, Clara) would have on my life.

I ended up studying with Mr. Pilates, and through a formal training program exclusively designed for me and Lolita San Miguel and administered through the State University of New York, I became certified to teach his methods. In 1972, I took over the Pilates studio located in Henri Bendels, a department store in midtown Manhattan, and I ran the studio from 1972 through 1988. During that time I created pre-Pilates warm-ups. My warm-ups gave the (mostly) women who took my classes a chance to transition from their hectic Superwoman Syndrome to the quiet concentration required to do Pilates. (The warm-ups also gave me a chance to pace the client flow in my small studio.)

When Jillian Hessel came to me in 1981, I remember saying to her, "I don't know what to do with you." Her back was so misaligned from years of rigorous ballet training that she couldn't even breathe properly. She didn't have much body and core strength, she had no abdominals, and her back muscles were completely imbalanced. So for want of something to occupy her time until I could figure out what to do with her crooked body, I started working with her on her breathing. Once she learned to breathe properly, we moved on to my warm-ups—which she really needed.

Jillian first came to me as a client and then became an apprentice teacher. She has now been teaching for 22 years and running a successful Los Angeles Pilates studio, the Well-Tempered Workout, since 1988. She has trained many teachers in Pilates since then. I feel that her coming to me as an injured dancer all those years ago has helped her to be a more inventive and patient teacher of Pilates exercise. Jillian had to work hard to get the concepts of Pilates into her body. She understands the potential fear, pain, and frustration of a beginning exerciser because she had to start over from the beginning to retrain her misaligned back. And although I can still spot Jillian's back condition, you may be hard pressed to find it. That's the power of Pilates.

You, the reader, stand to gain much from all Jillian has learned, not just from me, but from all of her movement teachers. I know she has continued to study—as all teachers must—in order to remain inspired.

I'm proud of Jillian for carrying on in the spirit of Joseph and Clara Pilates. She makes starting Pilates easy, fun, and nonthreatening with her B.E.A.M. Fundamentals. The Fundamentals will prepare any healthy beginning exerciser to perform classic Pilates matwork in the best way possible. I know this book will encourage you to move, look, and feel great.

And now, as I like to tell my students, "Get a move on!"

Kathleen Stanford-Grant (Kathy Grant)
Teacher of Pilates
New York University Tisch School of the Arts
New York, New York
November 2002

ACKNOWLEDGMENTS

I would like to thank so many folks for helping me to bring this book to fruition. First, there are my many students who have consistently said through the years that I should write a book. I was always flattered and thanked them, but secretly I wondered how I would ever find the time to pursue such an ambitious project. Then along came Andrea Lesky, my producer at Gaiam. He is a big-idea man, and if it weren't for his total belief in me and for the wonderful support system that has been created to help me along, you would not be holding this book in your hands.

Ron Derhacopian shot some gorgeous photos for the book, and Helen Jeffers, Sherri Berman, and Jetty Stutzman helped me to look good in the shots. Cheryl Montelle was my steadfast spotter who prompted me to "pull my ribs in." Cheryl also helped me to sort through, select, and arrange the hundreds of photos shot for this book. Mikael Salazar is a computer genius who helped me immeasurably with the technical writing of the exercise instruction and a rough draft of the instructional layout for the book. Kerry Eielson fleshed out the book's outline and did the initial writing of the first chapter.

My editors at Rodale Inc.—Margot Schupf and Christine Bucks—have been ever eager but extremely patient as I submitted materials to them well past the original deadlines. Joanna Williams has done a beautiful job bringing the book to life on the page.

Additional thanks must go to my husband, Arthur Spivak, for all his sage advice, and to my two children, Daniel and Miranda, who have had to put up with seeing less of me as I put in long hours at work to complete this project. Finally, I want to thank all the students I have taught over the past 22 years. It's from teaching you that I garnered the knowledge and experience to be able to write this book! I hope everyone feels as satisfied as I am that together we have created a completely unique and very valuable teaching tool that was worth waiting for.

PILATES: THE ROAD TO A NEW YOU

So you've heard about the Pilates (pih-LAH-teez) method of exercise, and you're intrigued. Perhaps you're attracted by some of its reported benefits, such as a long, lean, and supple body that moves with grace and style. But you wonder, Is Pilates really for *me*?

The answer, quite simply, is that Pilates is for everyone. In the following pages, you'll learn how to harness and develop your physical and mental abilities so that you'll find yourself moving better not only when you exercise, but during every task you perform throughout your day.

All of us are born with the potential for an endless variety of movement. And we all possess the inborn ability to move with natural grace as we go about our daily activities. The problem is that for most of us, exercise has become a necessary evil that we have to sandwich into our busy lives. We don't make time for it because we're too exhausted and stressed out after a day of work.

If you think you don't have time to exercise, then this is the book for you. It's also the book for you if you *do* exercise but are bored with your current program—or if you find you've reached a plateau and aren't getting the results you're looking for.

Whatever your reasons for buying this book and whatever your fitness level, get ready for a unique workout. Pilates builds from the ground up and gives you a whole new perspective on the hows and whys of the way your body moves. If you stick with it, Pilates will probably redefine your concept of what it means to be fit. It will uniformly strengthen muscles you never knew existed or mattered, and it will lengthen and smooth muscles you've given up hope on. It can realign your spine, flatten your stomach, improve your posture, and make you look and feel 10 years younger and 10 pounds lighter. In short, with regular practice, Pilates will make you feel as if you have a whole new body.

What Is *Pilates Basics*?

Just as the Pilates method of exercise is entirely unique, this book is different from all the other Pilates books you may find on the bookshelf. That's because it's for the Pilates novice—the person who has never practiced Pilates before.

In the first two chapters of *Pilates Basics,* you'll learn about the fundamentals of Pilates and how Joseph Pilates developed his method. You'll also learn how to assess your own posture and identify the all-important area of the body that Pilates called the Powerhouse.

In Chapter 3, you'll begin your workout with my B.E.A.M. Fundamentals (Breathe, Energize, Align, and Move). The Fundamentals prepare you for the classic Pilates matwork to come—sort of like learning to walk before you run. (Read more about the B.E.A.M. Fundamentals below.) Chapter 4 presents you with new challenges as you integrate all you've learned in the Fundamentals section into a more difficult routine based on Joseph Pilates's classic matwork series. I've rounded out the book with a bonus chapter of auxiliary exercises that will help you integrate your Pilates practice into your everyday activities. These exercises are great because you can do them in five minutes or less.

My Perspective on Pilates Today

I've been teaching Pilates since 1981, and I've had the good fortune to study with the absolute best of the first generation of teachers that Joseph Pilates trained: Kathleen Stanford-Grant, Carola Trier, Ron Fletcher, Eve Gentry, and Romana Kryszanowska. Kathy Grant and Eve Gentry were instrumental in introducing me to the idea of pre-Pilates warm-ups, as Kathy likes to call them. And Ron Fletcher has had an indelible influence on how I teach the use of breath control. I've found that all my students, young or old, fit or flabby, can benefit from learning my pre-Pilates warm-ups—the B.E.A.M. Fundamentals—before they tackle the classic matwork exercises.

Why? Well, when Pilates invented his original routines back in the 1930s, people were less stressed out and more active than they are today. Pilates workouts require body awareness, mental focus, and breath control. If we are disconnected from our bodies to begin with, how can we get centered enough to reap the full benefits of the method? I believe my B.E.A.M. Fundamentals are the answer.

These exercises begin with "B" for breathing, and as all yoga practitioners know, the breath can be a very powerful tool for quieting both the body and the mind. However, the breath can also invigorate you. By alternating slow, deep breaths with short, percussive breaths, you can consciously raise your body's energy level. And that leads to "E" for energy—which you obviously need if you're going to exercise! The "A" in B.E.A.M. is for alignment, as good form throughout your Pilates workout is vital. And of course, "M" is for move, because you'll learn to move dynamically in perfect form.

A Word to the Wise

As anyone can tell you, it takes time to master a new skill, and Pilates is no exception. Be patient with yourself, and don't become discouraged. It takes time to change your breathing and your posture, but the long-term benefits are well worth the effort. If you haven't been exercising regularly, make sure to check with your physician first, and start this program slowly.

Your Future Begins Now

The Pilates method may provide you with your first glimpse of your body's true potential for graceful movement, flexibility, and power. If you are committed, consistent, and patient, your hard work will pay off—and you'll be rewarded with a sense of calm that comes from living in a harmonious body, mind, and spirit. And now, as my teacher and mentor Carola Trier used to say, it's time to get going!

Jillian Hessel

Part One: Pilates Primer

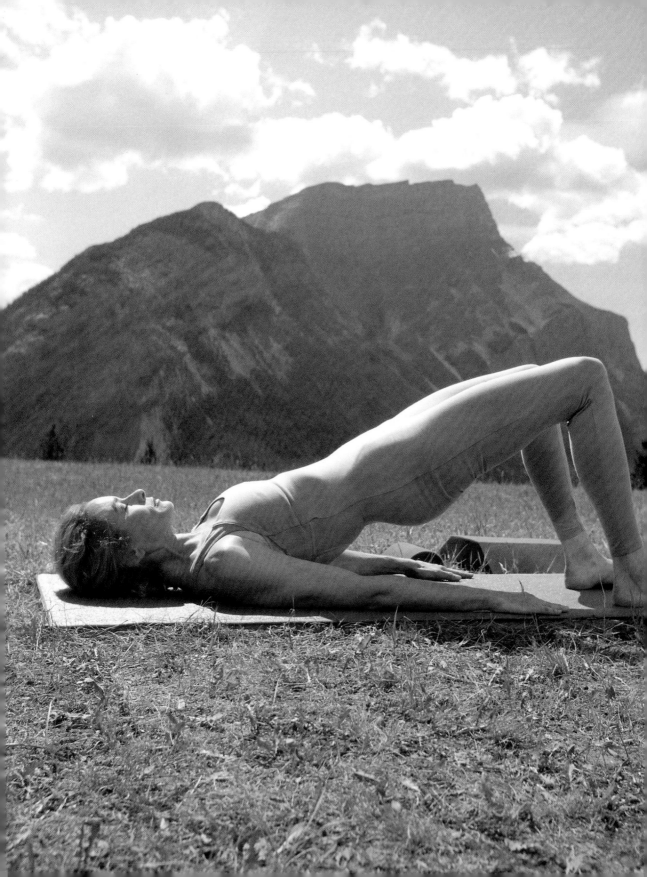

[1]

UNDERSTANDING THE NUTS
AND BOLTS

"There is no reason why each one of you can't experience your own body as beautiful no matter what your age, your shape, or how you feel about yourself now. That's what Body Contrology (the original name for Pilates exercise) is all about: learning more about your body, getting in better touch with all its parts and setting up a communication system with it, trusting and loving it as your best friend and then using it correctly all the time."

—**Ron Fletcher,** Pilates teacher who studied directly with Joseph and Clara Pilates from 1947 until 1971. He is widely recognized as a Master Teacher and is the founder of the Ron Fletcher Work.

WAKING UP YOUR BODY

As I mentioned in my introduction, Pilates is a form of exercise that's for everyone—young or old, fit or flabby. Like many other kinds of exercise, Pilates increases metabolism, promotes respiratory and circulatory function, and improves your bone density and muscle tone. Like yoga and martial arts, it can help you to "get centered" and calm your nerves. *Unlike* many other forms of exercise, however, Pilates balances out muscular asymmetries, streamlines your silhouette, and improves your balance, coordination, and breath control. Pilates does all this because the exercises work to simultaneously develop your muscular flexibility and your strength. The exercises also help you to awaken a new body awareness, or what I call your "inner eye."

With all that said, what makes Pilates so pertinent to the way you live your life today?

Well, Pilates is all about breathing and moving more fully—both of which we need to do more often. Over the last 50 years, our lifestyles have become increasingly sedentary, while our bodies, which were built for action, haven't changed in design.

We call sitting still for long periods of time "discipline," but it can be a kind of tyranny. If you sit at work or on an airplane for an extended time, you know how stiff and tired you can become. Getting up for a short stretch or a drink of water feels great, doesn't it? That's because you're satisfying your body's natural instinct to move—and moving around pumps more oxygen to your brain and your body.

The results of this immobile lifestyle are oxygen deprivation and disproportionate muscle development. Most of us walk around in a perpetually oxygen-deprived state. (No wonder we drink so much coffee.) In addition, being seated for long periods of time, combined

THE MAN BEHIND THE METHOD

Joseph Pilates was born in Germany in 1880 to parents of Greek ancestry. Small and sickly as a child, he became self-educated in anatomy, bodybuilding, wrestling, yoga, gymnastics, and martial arts. Pilates was enamored of the classical Greek ideal of a man who is balanced equally in body, mind, and spirit. He came to believe that our modern lifestyle, bad posture, and inefficient breathing were the roots of poor health. His answer to these problems was to design a unique series of vigorous physical exercises that help to correct muscular imbalances and improve posture, coordination, balance, strength, and flexibility, as well as to increase breathing capacity and organ function.

Pilates was touring England as a circus performer during World War I when he was interned as an enemy alien. He encouraged all his fellow prisoners to follow his exercise routines. However, some of the injured German soldiers were too weak to leave their beds. Not content to leave his comrades lying idle, Pilates took springs from the beds and attached them to the headboards and footboards of the iron bed frames, turning them into equipment that provided a type of resistance exercise for his bedridden "patients." These were the earliest models of the spring-based exercise apparatuses, such as the Cadillac and the Universal Reformer, for which the Pilates method is known today. Pilates legend has it that during the flu epidemic in 1918, not one of Pilates's "patients" died. He credited his technique with the prisoners' strength and fitness—remarkable under an internment camp's living conditions.

Pilates returned to Germany after the war, and his achievements with the German soldiers did not go unnoticed. In 1926, the German Kaiser invited him to begin training the German secret police. At this point, Pilates decided to emigrate to the United States. He met his future wife and dedicated teaching partner, Clara, on the boat to New York City. Together they opened the first Body Contrology (Pilates's name for his form of exercise) Studio on Eighth Avenue in Manhattan.

The earliest American students of Body Contrology were professional dancers, because they repeatedly injured themselves. Soon the choreographer George Balanchine and other movement visionaries became believers in Body Contrology. From there the exercise, but not the name, caught on—everyone seemed to prefer to call it Pilates. Today, many famous athletes, dancers, models, and actors—as well as business professionals, housewives, and retirees—have joined the ranks of Pilates practitioners.

with actions that require similar movements (such as writing, typing, driving, and eating), builds the muscles in the front of your upper body, making them strong and tight. These repetitive actions also stretch out the muscles in your upper back, making them long and weak. And of course, a slumping upper body only serves to further impair your breathing mechanism by closing down your chest, lungs, and diaphragm.

You don't have to end up hunched over and looking old before your time, though. (Two of my teachers and mentors, Kathy Grant and Ron Fletcher, are vigorous octogenarians, and they are still inspiring students and teaching them about the wonders of Pilates exercise.) Pilates is an education for your muscles—a primer on how they should be working all the time. Pilates teaches a consistent, concentrated way of combining deep, rhythmic breathing with movement. These exercises are so anatomically sound that they should extend into how you use your body every day. Whether you're getting out of a car, sitting at a desk, carrying a baby, walking your dog, or climbing stairs, your muscles will function at optimal capacity, holding your skeleton in proper alignment at all times. You'll find that everything you do reinforces Pilates, and vice versa.

And here's another big bonus of a Pilates workout: It doesn't require you to perform endless repetitions of boring, mindless exercises, and you won't suffer undue muscle strain, so there's little risk of injury. The emphasis in this type of exercise is on the ease and flow of movement, not on temple-popping exertion (although Pilates *is* mentally and physically challenging). Start with only 20-to-30-minute sessions two or three days a week. One precisely executed Pilates session is worth more than several hours at the gym—and you'll feel invigorated after Pilates, not worn out!

Moving from Your Core

The key to Pilates revolves around using the core of your body—what Joseph Pilates called the Powerhouse. Your body's center of gravity—

its core—is located approximately 2 inches below your navel. Pilates felt that all movements of the body should emanate from this power nexus. (This was a concept he borrowed from martial arts theory.) When the muscles of the Powerhouse are strong, your body can perform increasingly complex movements with balance, control, and ease. This is because you're working from where your body is most stable, rather than working from your body's periphery, as you do when a movement originates in your arms or legs.

A strong core is the reason that a thin, lean person like Bruce Lee can be more powerful than a muscle-bound bodybuilder. By the same token, a strong core is the reason a sumo wrestler, who looks incredibly unfit with all that fat, is nonetheless a pretty powerful guy.

Moving from the core also maximizes your energy. Think of the difference between a beginning and a professional figure skater. Beginners tend to flail their arms and bend over too far from the waist as they slip and slide across the ice. Professional skaters settle into their center of gravity and glide fluidly as they skate. Professionals might use their arms for artistic expression or to counterbalance a vigorous move, but all directional changes are made from the center of the torso and move down into their legs from the core of their bodies. Experienced skaters burn a lot fewer calories than beginners do and are much less fatigued by an hour of skating. That doesn't mean they're not getting a good workout, though, because this energy conservation means they'll have the endurance to continue skating for a much longer period of time than a beginner would.

The Art of Breathing Properly

Improving lung function and ensuring proper breathing technique should be the foundation of every Pilates session, simply because we don't ordinarily use our lungs to capacity. We are a world of shallow breathers. This means that most of us are using primarily our upper bodies, rather than our chest cavities, to breathe. We elevate our collarbones and upper shoulders, and we even tense our neck muscles when we inhale deeply. That doesn't do much good, though, since our lungs aren't located in our necks and there's no carbon dioxide/oxygen exchange in our shoulder muscles!

Shallow breathing can be the beginning of a downward spiral of health problems. It impairs mental acuity, causes headaches, increases anxiety, hampers the immune system, slows circulation, and decreases muscle and organ function. Lack of fresh oxygen in your system can also cause muscle cramps and an overall lack of vitality.

To breathe properly, you need to understand how your breathing mechanism is designed to work. When you inhale deeply, your diaphragm contracts and moves downward from your chest cavity into your abdominal cavity. The downward pull of the diaphragm creates a vacuum in your lungs, which causes them to fill up with fresh air. Muscles that run between your ribs, called intercostals, also contract to elevate your ribs, expanding your chest cavity to further increase your lung capacity.

When you exhale, the diaphragm relaxes and a different set of intercostals contracts to depress the ribs, causing the air to be expelled from your lungs. Pilates's groundbreaking idea was to increase the volume of air entering and exiting the lungs by not only strengthening the diaphragm and intercostal muscles, but also forcefully contracting the abdominals to aid each exhalation, thereby squeezing *all* the air from the lungs. The Pilates breath is intended to detoxify and invigorate. When we exhale completely, Pilates reasoned, we expel more toxins and carbon dioxide from the body and make room for the next inhalation, which should bring in as much fresh oxygen as possible. So with each new breath cycle, we purge the lungs of impurities and feed the brain and muscles fresh oxygen.

The milking action of deep abdominal contractions to boost the volume of air exhaled from the lungs is another factor that makes Pilates such a unique form of exercise. When you synchronize movement with breathing this way, you will automatically work from your core center, as Pilates intended. The combination of powerful breathing and carefully designed exercises will also provide an in-

THE BODY-MIND CONNECTION

Unless you're familiar with yoga, meditation, or the martial arts, the body-mind connection may be a completely new concept to you. What is it? The body-mind connection is simply a way of becoming more aware, or mindful, of your actions. The goal is to fully experience what is going on in the present moment—nothing more and nothing less. When you're practicing Pilates, this means you're aware of not only the movements that you're doing, but also the quality of those movements and how they're timed with the rhythm of your breath.

The body-mind connection is the key to reducing stress in our lives. The "fight or flight" reaction to danger in the wild that pumped our ancestors full of adrenaline to ensure their survival still works the same for us. However, when you become frustrated sitting in a traffic jam or have a tough day at the office or with the kids, you usually can't fight or run away. If a safe, acceptable physical outlet for your frustration isn't available, the hormones from the adrenaline rush stay in your system. Your blood pressure rises, your heart rate speeds up, your immune system is depressed, and you become more stressed out.

The body-mind connection helps you gain control of your nervous system. Learning to calm down and work from your core can help you to find a safe and healthy way to get rid of everyday stress and tension. And since Pilates is a form of body-mind exercise, you'll reap mental benefits as well as physical ones from it.

The body-mind connection begins with breath, which you can learn all about in "Setting the Foundation: B.E.A.M. Fundamentals," beginning on page 48.

ternal massage for your vital organs, stimulating circulation and digestion. And of course, strengthening the abdominals creates strong support for your back. So when you perform a thorough, concentrated Pilates session, you're not only improving your lung capacity and expelling toxins from your body; you're also improving your posture and flattening your stomach!

After just a few days of breathing more consciously, you'll find you feel more energized and alive. Just being aware of your breath will make a huge difference in your health and quality of life.

Increasing Your Flexibility

Some people actually think stretching is a waste of time because they believe flexibility isn't important and doesn't do anything to improve the way they look. Nothing could be further from the truth! Flexibility is an integral part of Pilates, and Pilates exercises are unique because they combine building muscle strength with increasing muscle flexibility.

Flexibility increases your range of motion, which will help to prevent injuries, and also helps to restore correct alignment to your bone structure. Stretching soothes sore muscles, eases chronic pain, and relieves nervous tension. Improved flexibility visibly lengthens muscles over time and will make you look and feel taller, leaner, younger, and more toned. In contrast, overdeveloping your muscles without stretching makes your body look compact, as if your muscles are packed on your frame like handfuls of clay.

Stretching also helps to increase blood flow to your muscles. The act of alternately lengthening and relaxing a muscle as you stretch flushes blood and toxins, such as lactic acid and carbon dioxide, out and allows freshly oxygenated blood to flow back in. Combined with deep breathing, stretching is a powerful component to becoming more fit, because a stretched muscle is toned, invigorated, and ready to move in any direction.

Fitness Redefined

Throw out the notion that you have to go for the burn during your Pilates sessions in order to become fit. Fitness is not about doing hardcore workouts that bust your gut every time. Soreness is not a sign that you've had a good workout; it's a sign that you've overworked your muscles to the extent that they are unable to function. Exercise shouldn't hurt—during or after the workout.

You don't have to sweat buckets, overheat, or exercise until you're red in the face to purge toxins from your body and raise your metabolism.

INVEST THE TIME

Time will always be an issue, so it's up to you to make the most of yours when it comes to exercising. Don't cheat yourself. Making time for exercise is fundamental to keeping your body and mind healthy. Regular exercise is not only about looking good; it's also about putting a premium on how you feel. It's about being strong, graceful, and alive and functioning at your best—physically and mentally. Wouldn't it be foolish to waste your most important assets—your health and well-being?

Exercise is worth doing for even short periods of time. If you don't have a full hour, try doing a half hour or even 15 minutes of exercise. Do what you can to fit exercise in with your lifestyle. Pilates sessions will help you with this, because the Pilates mindset encourages you to become aware of how you use your body all the time—not just when you're exercising. Also, be sure to take a look at "Take 5: Auxiliary Exercises," beginning on page 136. There you'll find some great suggestions on how to integrate Pilates into everyday life in quick five-minute routines.

Huffing and puffing is not the only way to improve respiration, lower stress, and improve circulation. Controlled deep breathing works just as well, or better, both to detoxify and to give you an exercise high.

Finally, a good Pilates session shouldn't tire you out. It should energize and invigorate both your mind and body, not push them to the point of exhaustion. Aren't you ready for a change?

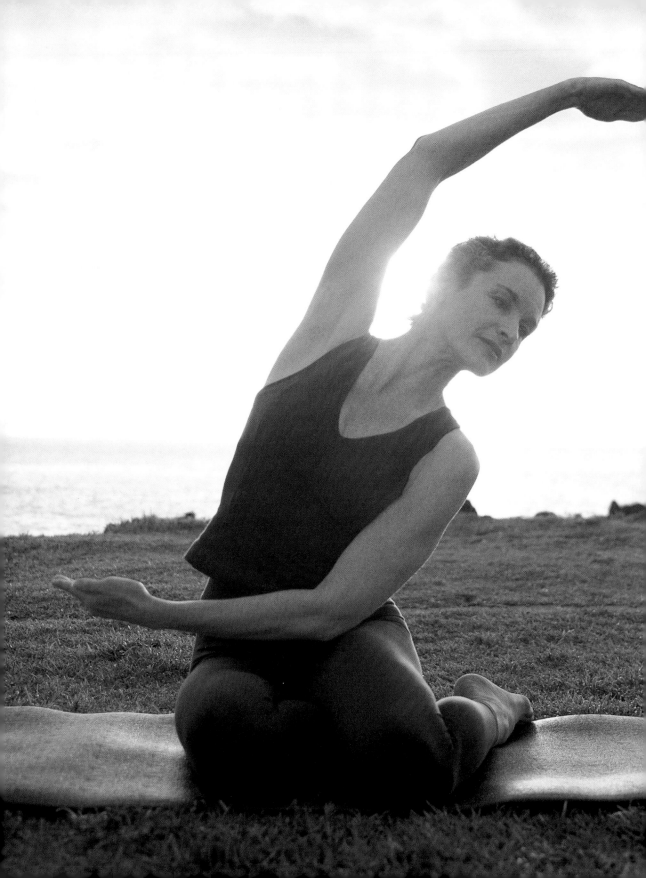

[2]

PERFECTING YOUR POSTURE

Good posture is taught by military academies, modeling agencies, dancing schools, and everyone's mother. Why? Because a person who moves well in her body projects a sense of power, grace, self-confidence, and personal style. If your posture is equivalent to a lazy slump, you'll end up with a thick waist, narrow chest, and rounded shoulders that make you look at least 2 inches shorter—definitely not the picture of grace and style! Good posture is about more than just looking good, though; it's essential for a healthy, well-functioning body.

Poor posture is an energy sapper. If your spine is incorrectly balanced, your muscles need to work harder to keep your body upright all day long. Lazy posture also causes your upright structure to collapse in places, like a poorly constructed building. This collapsed structure can compound many physical ailments, including constipation and other digestive problems, poor circulation, chronic low energy, lower back pain, headaches, and shortness of breath.

Standing tall may feel more tiring at first because you'll have to retrain and strengthen the core muscles in your body to improve your posture. However, once you've begun using the B.E.A.M. Fundamentals presented in this book (see Chapter 3, beginning on page 48), you'll never forget the basic principles of support, breath work, and movement. You'll move with more grace and power, not just when you're exercising, but throughout your day. And you'll be amazed at how much more energy you'll have!

THE SKINNY ON YOUR SPINE

The human spine is made up of 32 to 34 bones called vertebrae. The spine is constructed to provide a maximum range of motion and support for the body with a minimum of wear and tear on the spine's joints, or intervertebral discs. The discs lie between the vertebrae, and they provide cushioning that helps to reduce friction in the joints when you move.

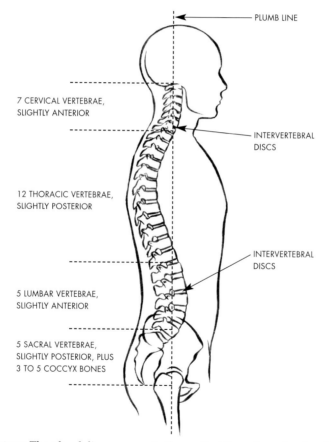

PLUMB LINE

7 CERVICAL VERTEBRAE, SLIGHTLY ANTERIOR

INTERVERTEBRAL DISCS

12 THORACIC VERTEBRAE, SLIGHTLY POSTERIOR

INTERVERTEBRAL DISCS

5 LUMBAR VERTEBRAE, SLIGHTLY ANTERIOR

5 SACRAL VERTEBRAE, SLIGHTLY POSTERIOR, PLUS 3 TO 5 COCCYX BONES

Ideal posture: The plumb line represents the vertical line of gravity that falls through your body. When properly aligned, the line enters directly through the crown of your head and bisects the cervical curve. It then travels through the center of your chest cavity and bisects the center of the lumbar curve. Finally, it passes through the center of the pelvis and hip joint. This is a spine in ideal alignment and is called physiologically efficient posture.

The spine has four natural curves—three flexible and one fixed. In a side view of the body, the normal curves in an ideal posture appear as follows:

* A forward, or anterior, curve in the 7 cervical vertebrae that form your neck.

* A backward, or posterior, curve in the 12 thoracic vertebrae, where the ribs attach to form your upper torso.

* Another anterior curve in the 5 lumbar vertebrae that form your lower back.

* A final posterior curve in the 5 fused bones of the sacrum, where your pelvis attaches to your spine. This curve is completed by 3 to 5 coccyx bones, also fused, that form your tailbone.

The first three curves of the body are flexible, which means that this is where you bend and twist your spine. However, the sacral/coccygeal curve is fixed, since the vertebrae there are fused.

If your mom always told you to stand up straight, she was wrong! The spinal curves lend shock absorption, extra flexibility, and range of motion to your movement, so you don't want to flatten them out or eliminate them. You *can* run into structural problems and back pain, however, if there is too much or too little curve in your spine, or if the curves do not balance properly with one another.

The degree of spinal curve may vary from person to person, but the key here is that the curves of each individual must balance with one another within that person's particular body type in order to achieve ideal posture. Good posture can help us to attain (and retain as we age) maximum flexibility, strength, resiliency, and mobility of the spine. This is a goal well worth aiming for, and regular Pilates workouts can help you achieve it because postural awareness is built right in to every exercise.

Posture and Your Back

Poor posture results in misaligned vertebrae and either an exaggeration or a flattening of the natural curves of the spine. These poorly aligned postures cause asymmetrical muscle development, meaning certain muscle groups are constantly overworking to hold the body upright while others become significantly weakened. Poor posture makes the body more injury-prone because the intervertebral discs are under constant stress from the misalignments. In addition, uneven development of the back muscles combined with weak abdominal support can be an accident waiting to happen. For example, many people injure their backs when they make a simple but abrupt movement, such as bending to pick up an item dropped on the floor or twisting to reach something in the backseat of a car. Having evenly developed back muscles and strong abs can help you avoid such injuries.

Even our favorite sports, such as golf, tennis, and running, encourage lopsided and uneven muscle development—as does carrying a briefcase or handbag on one side of your body or balancing an infant on the same hip for hours and hours.

Pilates can be a wonderful solution to all these poor postural habits because the exercises encourage bilateral, even muscle development and flexibility at the same time. A good Pilates workout doesn't have to be long or exhausting, but it can and will rebalance your body over time.

Problem Postures

Problem postures come in an endless variety, but over the next two pages I've defined the big four—the most common problems.

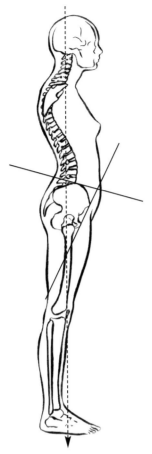

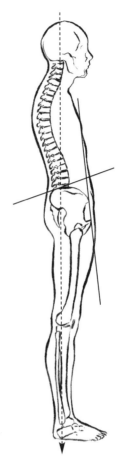

Kyphosis/Lordosis. This posture exhibits an exaggerated rounding of the upper back and shoulders along with a forward head and overarched lower back. People who stand like this often suffer from lower back pain and mistakenly blame their discomfort solely on weak back muscles. This is simply not the case. In this posture, the neck extensors (muscles in the back of the neck), lower back, and hip flexor muscles (the muscles that cross the front of the hip joint) are extremely strong and tight. The abs and upper back muscles, on the other hand, are weak and splayed out. You can correct this posture by stretching out the tight muscles in the neck, lower back, and hip flexors, and by strengthening the abs and upper back muscles.

Swayback syndrome. In this posture, the knees are locked backward and the pelvis is tucked under, which has the effect of flattening out the natural curve in the lower back. The shoulders round forward and the chest caves in as the chin juts forward. This posture is common among teenage boys who want to look cool, but also has become more prevalent among adults with sedentary jobs. As in the Kyphosis/Lordosis posture, the neck extensors must be stretched to lengthen the back of the neck, and the upper back muscles must be strengthened to lessen the upper back curve. However, the hamstrings (the muscles in the backs of the thighs) are short in this posture and should be stretched in order to allow the pelvis to release to a more neutral position.

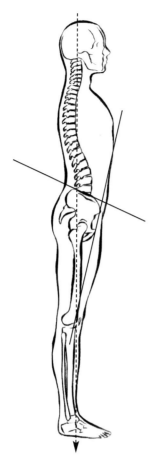

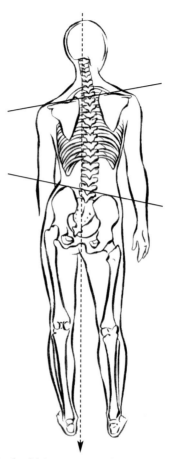

Military posture. This posture is the classic look we assume when trying too hard to stand up straight. The chest pops out in front and the head is held at attention, resulting in extreme rigidity in the upper back and neck. The lower back is overarched, as in the Kyphosis/ Lordosis posture, and the knees are locked backward. People who stand this way suffer from allover stiffness and a limited range of motion. I recommend an overall stretching program that emphasizes breathing and relaxation, as well as specific stretching to lengthen the muscles of the lower back and hip flexors.

Cocked-hip posture. This is a typically feminine stance, and this form of femininity has its price: imbalanced muscles that are weak on one side and strong on the other. One shoulder is often higher than the other, and the torso rotates clockwise or counterclockwise so that one hip or shoulder is more forward than the other. Needless to say, this posture is not efficient in terms of weight-bearing exercise or stability. I recommend a good overall stretching and strengthening program, with specific attention paid to stretching the tight muscles on one side of the body and strengthening the weak muscles on the other side in order to balance out the overall posture.

CHECKING YOUR OWN POSTURE

I always take my first-time clients through a fitness interview and then do a postural evaluation before we begin learning the B.E.A.M. Fundamentals. I like to do this because I can learn a lot by observing a person in the posture she walks around in all day. After all, if the eventual goal is to stand up straighter or tone certain muscle groups, it's helpful for both the client and me to acknowledge our starting-off point, which will help us to set realistic long-term goals.

It just makes sense to include a posture self-check in this book to aid you in your self-assessment and goal-setting processes. As you progress in your Pilates workouts, it may be helpful for you to return to this section from time to time to reevaluate yourself and check for improvement.

Ideally, you should perform this posture check standing in front of a mirror. To make the process easier, read this part of the book aloud into a tape recorder and play it back while you evaluate yourself. If a mirror evaluation is not an option, ask a friend to check your posture, and then check hers.

WHAT TO WEAR

When assessing your own posture, make sure you wear comfortable but form-fitting clothing so that you can see your body and imagine its underlying bone structure. (Loose clothing can hide a multitude of problems.) Take off your socks and shoes so you can see your feet. If your pants are baggy, roll them up so you can see your ankles and knees. If your T-shirt is oversized, tuck it into your pants. Finally, if you have long hair, tie it up off your neck so you become aware of how you carry your head.

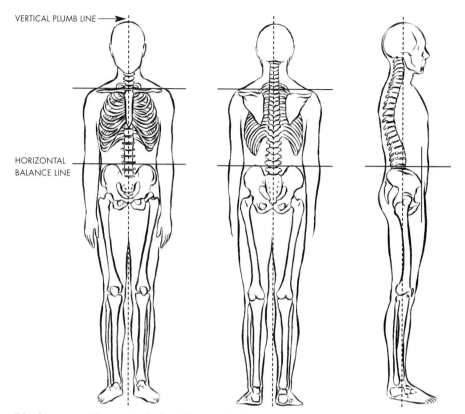

VERTICAL PLUMB LINE →

HORIZONTAL
BALANCE LINE

Ideal posture: The vertical plumb line in the front and back views is a means to measure body symmetry from left to right. The horizontal lines run parallel to one another and show the shoulders and hips in balanced alignment. Compare this to the cocked-hip posture on page 30. In the side view, the vertical line in front of the pelvis denotes a level or neutral pelvis. Observe how it intersects the horizontal line drawn at the top of the pelvis at a 90-degree angle, and compare this to the faulty postures shown on pages 29 and 30.

Your Feet—The Foundation

Let's begin with your feet. One of my mentors, Carola Trier, used to say, "So you say your back hurts? Let me see your feet." That's because your feet are the foundation of your entire upright structure. Think of your body as a building, with your feet as the foundation on which you build the upper stories. If something is out of alignment in the foundation of your building, the upper stories will mirror that imbalance in an attempt to balance your unsteady structure. This is why misaligned feet really *can* affect your back.

Put your hands on your hipbones in the front of your pelvis and align your feet directly under your hip sockets. Lift your toes off the floor and spread them apart like you're opening a fan. Place your toes on the floor, spreading your weight evenly across your forefeet. Rock forward and backward from toes to heels, and then settle your weight in the center of your foot. Roll your feet inward, then outward, and settle back to center.

Each foot should feel like a three-legged stool, with equal weight placed on the big toe, little toe, and heel.

Your Legs

Continuing with our building analogy, feel your legs rising up as the twin columns of your building. Keeping the tripod of each foot firmly rooted to the floor and your heels on the floor, do a small knee bend. Watch to see where your kneecaps go in relation to your feet. This is called "tracking," and ideally your bent knees should track directly over the center of your toes, between your second and third toes (see Fig. 1 below).

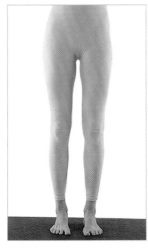

FIG. 1

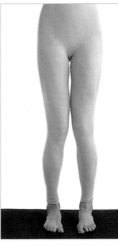

FIG. 2

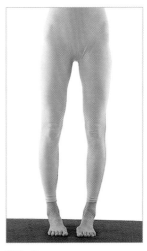

FIG. 3

If your kneecaps are tracking over your big toes, you're knock-kneed and probably somewhat flat-footed. This stance places a lot of stress on the inner side (medial portion) of your knee joint and can result in uneven wear and tear on the joint (see Fig. 2 on page 33). The opposite problem, where the knees track over the little toe, is less common but just as troublesome. It can be found in people with bunion pain in the big toe or in folks who are bowlegged (see Fig. 3 on page 33).

Now stand facing sideways to the mirror. Bend and straighten your knees once again, and look at the vertical line of your legs when they're straight. Are your knees still knobby? If so, your quadriceps (the muscles on the fronts of your thighs) are weak. Do your legs overstraighten into a locked-backward, or hyperextended, position? Hyperextended knees not only place undue pressure on your knee joints, but also affect the entire balance of your pelvis, as your body must compensate somewhere else for the leg misalignment.

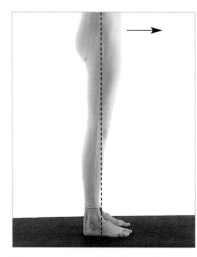

Correct posture: Ideal leg alignment with headlights pointing straight ahead.

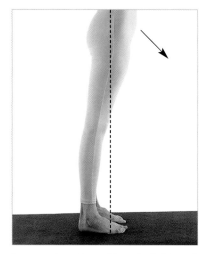

Incorrect posture: Overstraightened or hyperextended leg alignment causes the low back to overarch and headlights to tilt down.

The Bridge of the Pelvis

Returning to our building metaphor, the twin columns of your legs insert into your pelvis at your thigh sockets—making your pelvis a bridge between the upper and lower stories of your building. To reinforce your bridge and form a firm support for your spine, you need strong pelvic floor muscles, which you can achieve by performing Kegel exercises. Try isolating the pelvic floor muscles as often as you can by pulling them upward against gravity—as if you have a full bladder and are trying to stop the flow of urine. Because the work is all internal, you can practice Kegels when you're riding in an elevator, standing in a grocery store line, or driving your car.

For added support in your vertical posture, as well as for aesthetic reasons, it's important to have strong buttocks muscles. Pay particular attention to the base of your buttocks, where the backs of your thighs insert into your pelvis. I call the underside of the buttocks the "smile" muscles, because they should form a pleasing U shape under each buttock. To locate your smile muscles, imagine a bolt extending from the outside of one of your buttocks to the outside of the other, and tighten it.

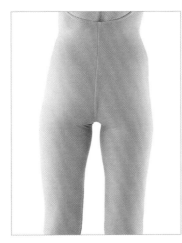

Smile muscles relaxed

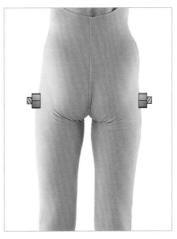

Smile muscles "bolted," or engaged

Neutral Pelvis Position

Next, let's find neutral pelvis position, which is the safest position for your lower back when you're bending or lifting. Place the heels of your hands on your hipbones at the front of your pelvis, and imagine your hipbones are the headlights on a car. When you're in neutral, your headlights shine straight out in front of you, and you can clearly see the road ahead (see Fig. 1 below). However, if your headlights shine downward, your lower back will overarch, and you won't be able to see much of the road (see Fig. 2 below). Conversely, if you tilt your headlights upward, your lower back loses its natural curve—and you certainly won't be able to drive very far (see Fig. 3 below)!

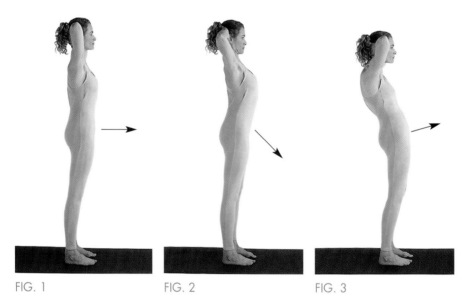

FIG. 1   FIG. 2   FIG. 3

Play around with balancing your headlights by overarching and tucking your pelvis back and forth until you come naturally to your best neutral position. Notice that your lower abdominals must engage to hold the neutral position. Now reinforce neutral by engaging your pelvic floor and smile muscles, too!

The Abs—Your Girdle of Strength

Joseph Pilates called the abs the girdle of strength because the abdominal muscles really do wrap around your torso like a girdle. And once you've learned to use your abs properly, you can throw away your artificial girdle forever, because you won't need it!

Your body has four different layers of abs, similar to the layers of an onion. The first and deepest layer is called the transverse abdominals. Their primary function is to contract forcefully when you exhale deeply, such as when you cough or sneeze. When the transverse abs contract, your lower belly should flatten. I call this action "scooping your abs." You can practice scooping by imagining you have a belt slung low across your hips, from hipbone to hipbone. Inhale deeply through your nose, and as you exhale through your mouth, imagine you're tightening the hip belt one notch tighter and drawing your hipbones closer together, maintaining the neutral position of the pelvis (see Fig. 1 below).

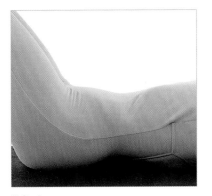 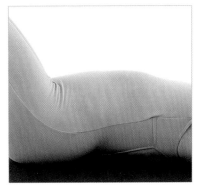

FIG. 1   FIG. 2

The opposite action of scooping is "pooching your abs," and many people who begin Pilates training find they've inadvertently trained the transverse abs to pooch rather than scoop (see Fig. 2 above). Be patient with yourself and continue to practice the B.E.A.M. Fundamentals, and this, too, shall pass.

The second and third layers of abdominals are called the internal and external obliques, and they run on opposite diagonals across the front of your body. I like to visualize two triangles drawn on the front of the torso. The first triangle uses the horizontal line between the hipbones as its base, with the point touching the navel. The second triangle is inverted, with its point also touching the navel, but its base stretches horizontally across the front of the rib cage (see Fig. 1 below). To engage your obliques, exhale once again, and imagine the points of your two triangles intersecting and then overlapping slightly (see Fig. 2 below).

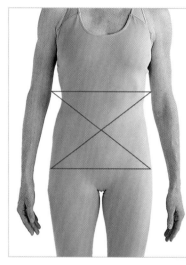

FIG. 1

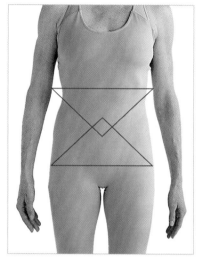

FIG. 2

The fourth and most superficial layer of abdominals is the rectus abdominis. This muscle runs vertically from your pubic bone all the way up to your breastbone. The rectus is considered a "vanity" muscle by body builders, who take pride in having a perfectly formed "six-pack." I like to think of zipping up a very tight pair of jeans or a jumpsuit to engage the rectus.

The Pilates Powerhouse

As I mentioned in Chapter 1, the Pilates method is based on the concept that all body movements should emanate from a strong and centered Powerhouse. The Powerhouse consists of the pelvic floor, "smile" muscles, and lower abdominal muscles, plus the lower back muscles. Your Powerhouse works when all of these muscles contract simultaneously. (This is called a co-contraction.) And the most supportive way for you to lift or bend, as well as to perform the exercises presented in this book, is by engaging your Powerhouse, so you'll definitely want to work to properly execute this concept.

To identify your Powerhouse, place the palm of one hand on the front of your lower abdomen and the palm of your other hand on your lower back. Inhale deeply through your nose, and exhale out through your mouth, pulling your lower abs up and in toward your backbone. Exhale completely, and your hands will come closer together as your waist gets thinner. Pilates called this action "navel to spine." Practice navel to spine several times, and then add the support of your pelvic floor, zipper, hip belt, and smile muscles at the same time. Congratulations—you've just identified your Powerhouse!

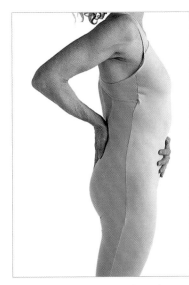

Inhale—Powerhouse relaxed

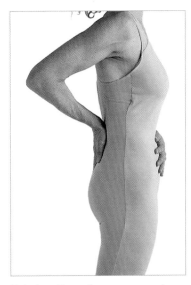

Exhale—Powerhouse engaged

The Upper Stories of Your Building

Floating above your Powerhouse are the upper stories of your building, consisting of your rib cage, chest, shoulders, neck, and head. It's easy to see how misalignments in your lower body are reflected and balanced out by more posture problems as you move up your spine. Tight upper back, shoulder, and neck muscles can cause tension headaches, while the round-shouldered look definitely makes a person look older. And of course, as I've mentioned before, poor posture can sap your energy.

Take a look again at the ideal and misaligned postures from the side view (see pages 26, 29, and 30), and this time note the vertical placement of the shoulders, neck, and head. In ideal alignment, the shoulder joints are in a straight vertical line over the hip joints, and the earlobes float vertically over the shoulder joints. When the head is properly balanced on the spine, the line of the jawbone is perpendicular to the throat.

Let's return to the image of the two triangles in the front of your torso merging together as you exhale. Turn sideways to a mirror while you do this, and notice that engaging the obliques can actually improve your posture by moving your shoulders into a more vertical line over your hips.

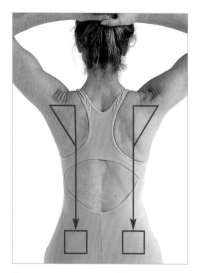

Correct shoulder position

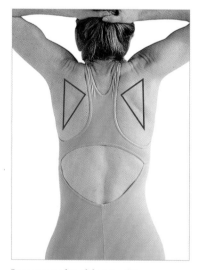

Incorrect shoulder position

Now imagine the flat triangle-shaped bones of your shoulder blades hugging the back of your rib cage. Notice how visualizing this image begins to open up the front of your shoulders. Inhale, and as you exhale, draw the lower points of your shoulder blades down your back and visualize them sliding into your back pockets (see the correct shoulder position on the opposite page). Don't let the triangles in the front of your body become separated! Allow your arms to relax and hang freely at your sides.

Now nod your head "yes." Gradually balance your head on top of your spine, focusing on lengthening the muscles at the back of your neck. Level your eyes straight ahead in this new posture, and scan your entire body once more. Hold on to your Powerhouse but release any excess tension.

Simultaneously feel your connection to the earth through the tripods of your feet and imagine that you are suspended by a giant marionette string from the crown of your head to the ceiling. I call this kind of imagery "two-way energy" because it causes you to lengthen in opposite directions simultaneously.

Maintaining two-way energy and the focus of your eyes, test your balance by rising onto the balls of your feet. Keep your weight balanced across your forefeet (see Fig. 1 below), and avoid rolling out or in (see Figs. 2 and 3 below). If your entire body is falling forward or backward as you try to balance, it's telling you that your posture is still not balanced correctly.

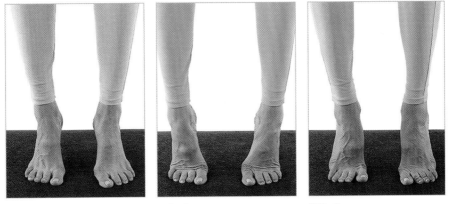

FIG. 1   FIG. 2   FIG. 3

POSTURE TIPS

Keep these additional tips in mind to help you maintain proper posture throughout your day:

☀ Carry a backpack instead of a shoulder bag; if you must carry a shoulder bag, switch shoulders daily to avoid becoming lopsided.

☀ Don't cross your legs while you sit.

☀ Take your wallet out of your back pocket before you sit down.

☀ Use a display rack to hold papers directly over your computer screen. If that's not an option, make sure to alternate which side of the keyboard you put your documents on so that your head isn't always turning in the same direction.

☀ Replace worn soles on your shoes.

☀ If you wear heels, alternate the shape and height of your shoes from day to day, and be aware that high heels tend to overarch your lower back.

☀ Carry your baby in a baby carrier or sling so that you're not hunching up one shoulder and hip to support the full weight of the baby. If you don't have a carrier, alternate hips whenever possible.

☀ Bend from your legs—not your back—when you bend over or lift a heavy object.

☀ Keep your spine reinforced in neutral alignment at all times by using the muscles of your Powerhouse.

☀ Exhale as you lift an object, keeping the object close to your core center as you carry it.

Still feeling the marionette string suspending you up through the crown of your head, slowly lower your heels back to the floor. You should feel taller and lighter than when you began.

How to Sit

So far in this chapter I've talked about ideal standing posture. But what happens to your spine when you sit down—especially on the floor, as opposed to in a chair? Do you tend to slump and collapse? Does a tight lower back or inflexible hips and short hamstrings prevent you from sitting up straight?

Because many Pilates mat exercises and our breathing practice in B.E.A.M. Fundamentals begin with you "sitting up tall," it's worth your time to experiment with props so that you can sit comfortably on your mat for a period of time. Take a look at the photos below showing a seated cross-legged position. You may notice a similarity to some of the poor postures we're already looked at.

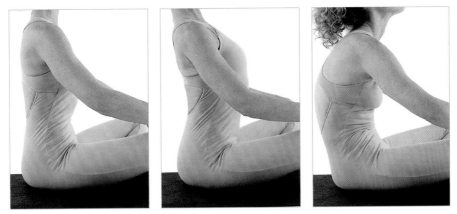

Good sitting posture   Seated military posture   Seated swayback posture

Quite often I see students have relatively good standing posture as well as good posture while seated in a chair, but they can't sit up tall when sitting on the floor on a mat. This lack of flexibility prevents good alignment of the spine and definitely inhibits a mastery of the Pilates matwork. So what do you do if you're one of these folks?

Try stacking up folded bath towels, firm blankets, or pillows to create a little throne for yourself. Put your buttocks on the throne, but leave your ankles on the floor. It isn't important how high or low your throne is, but in general, the more inflexible you are, the higher it should be. Make it just high enough so you can sit up tall out of your hips and elongate your spine. (Remember the image of the marionette string, and feel yourself being pulled upward.)

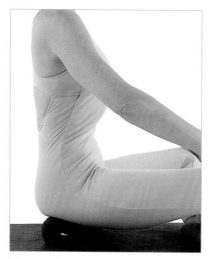

Use a cushion to achieve good posture.

If you're still feeling discomfort in your hip sockets because they're stretching when you sit this way, experiment with placing pillows or towels under your knees so they're supported in this position. As you become more flexible, you may find that you can gradually reduce the height of your supports—and one day you may not need them at all. However, please remember that the important thing is for you to feel comfortable and tall when sitting; that way, you can properly execute the breathing and exercise instructions.

That does it for my lesson on posture. Now that you know the components of proper standing and sitting posture—and have had a chance to evaluate your own posture—it's time to start working that body. So let's move on to the next chapter, where you'll find my pre-Pilates warm-ups: the B.E.A.M. Fundamentals.

GETTING STARTED

Before you start the exercises in the B.E.A.M. Fundamentals, keep the following points in mind:

* Make sure you don't have any health problems that preclude your doing these exercises.

* If you're pregnant or out of shape or have never exercised, please talk to your doctor before beginning this—or any—exercise program.

* Wait at least a half hour between eating a meal and starting your session.

* Make sure you've had plenty to drink so you're hydrated, and be sure that you feel well rested.

* Wear comfortable but somewhat form-fitting clothing so you can see and feel your body working in proper alignment.

* If you have long hair, tie it back away from your face.

* Make sure you have enough space within which to exercise. You'll need enough room to lie down with your arms stretched vertically over your head. If you find your arms or legs are running into walls or furniture, you'll need to pick an alternative workout space.

* Before you begin, gather a few props to use during the exercises: a padded surface or mat to lie on; a medium- to heavyweight, yard-long (or longer) exercise band; and firm pillows or folded towels. Start with at least one large folded bath towel to sit on and a smaller hand towel that you can fold or roll to support your head and neck when lying down. You can always add more props later or eliminate them as you see fit.

Part Two: Your Body in Motion

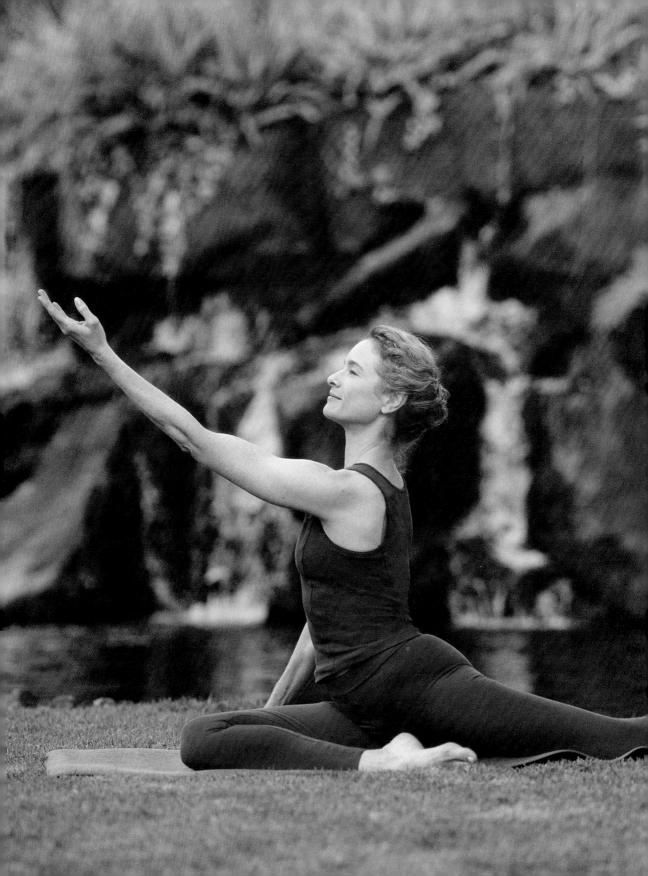

[3]

SETTING THE FOUNDATION: B.E.A.M. FUNDAMENTALS

Just as your feet are the foundation for good upright posture, the B.E.A.M. Fundamentals are the foundation for your Pilates practice. These preparatory exercises will help you warm up both body and mind, and enhance your understanding and execution of the more challenging classic matwork exercises to come in the next chapter.

As I explained in my introduction, B.E.A.M. is an acronym that stands for Breathe, Energize, Align, and Move. Since "B" is for Breathe, naturally you'll begin by observing how your breath travels in and out of your body. Next you'll establish conscious control of your breath, making it more dynamic to Energize (the "E" in B.E.A.M.) your entire body and mind. And you'll increase your understanding of the body-mind connection by engaging your deepest abdominal muscles, or "girdle of strength," and your pelvic floor muscles to initiate each exhalation.

To incorporate "A" for Align, you'll learn to visualize your bone structure, which supports all your body's movements. If you can visualize the best alignment of your bone structure before you begin a movement, your movements will be more efficient and less stressful on your body.

The "M" for Move is the final element of B.E.A.M. You'll find that applying your new knowledge of breath, energy, and alignment into dynamic movement is an exciting experience, whether it's for Pilates, competitive sports, or simply a walk around the block.

HELPFUL HINTS

The B.E.A.M. acronym appears alongside each exercise description to provide a quick overview of the following:

＊ *Breathe* gives the breathing pattern for the exercise.

＊ *Energize* suggests the mental imagery or visualizations you should keep in mind as you perform the exercise.

＊ *Align* lists important alignment pointers for each exercise.

＊ *Move* shows a pictorial progression of what the exercise should look like in motion, from start to finish.

The B.E.A.M. Fundamentals are designed to be a progression, meaning each new exercise builds on the skills you learned in the previous exercise. Take your time to learn each of the fundamentals individually and in the order in which I've presented them. Don't move on to the next exercise until you've thoroughly mastered the previous one. Taking the time to master each exercise will help you build a strong Powerhouse, promote more efficient breath control, and most important, help develop strong, graceful, flowing movement.

Note: There is one exception to learning the B.E.A.M. Fundamentals in the exact order presented here. When you come to Back Extensions (see page 78), you have the option of substituting the Airplane exercise (see page 80) for the Back Extensions. I've presented two different options for strengthening the muscles of your back because not everyone is comfortable lying on their stomachs for an extended period of time, as is called for in Back Extensions. The Airplane is a wonderful alternative back extensor exercise done on all fours. If you do choose the Airplane option, please remember to do Elbow Push-Ups first, as a preparatory exercise.

As you begin the exercises, you'll see I've included descriptions of how *not* to perform certain techniques in each exercise in a sidebar called "Body Scan." I've made these incorrect techniques easy for you to find by wearing a dark blue leotard in all of the "Body Scan" photos.

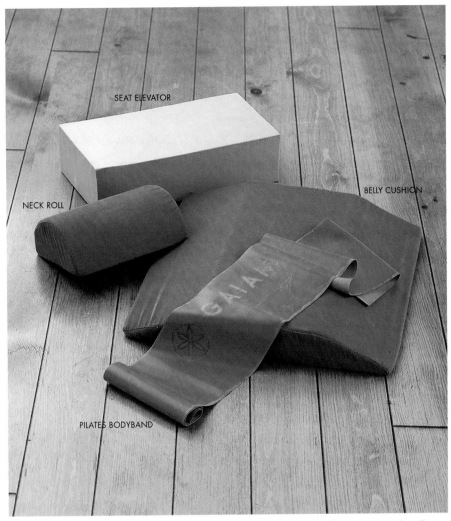

The Pilates basics props referenced in this book include a seat elevator, a neck roll, a belly cushion for extra support when lying on your stomach, and a Pilates BodyBand.

Of course, you may wish to gather your own props together using towels, blankets, or throw cushions from your home. Either way, use your props creatively and be responsive to your body's needs as you see fit. Your Pilates workouts will be that much more enjoyable and effective.

SEATED BREATHING

Of course, your workout must begin with controlled breath work. Pilates exercises are rhythmic, but we use no music, so breath control is vital for correct execution of the exercises. You'll focus here on two types of breathing: slow, deep breathing, and short, percussive breathing. These different breathing patterns will help you to accent the correct dynamics for each exercise.

BREATHE

Inhale through your nose, and exhale through your mouth. Move the largest volume of air possible in and out of your lungs with each breath.

ENERGIZE

Visualize your rib cage expanding horizontally like an accordion as you inhale. Initiate exhalation by visualizing your zipper, hip belt, navel to spine, and triangles.

ALIGN

In the upright posture (see Fig. 3), align your shoulders squarely over your hips, and feel yourself growing taller with each exhalation.

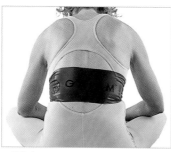
FIG. 1

FIG. 1

✳ To begin, wrap an exercise band around your rib cage and tie the ends in front. Round your back over to open up the back of your lungs. Exhale all the air. As you exhale, engage your zipper and draw your navel to spine.

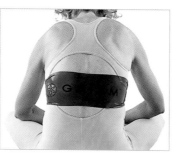
FIG. 2

FIG. 2

✳ Inhale deeply through your nose, concentrating on expanding the band to the back and sides of your rib cage. (Notice the letters on the band stretch farther apart on inhalation.) Avoid raising your shoulders or tensing your neck as you inflate your lungs like a balloon. Allow your ribs and exercise band to relax as you exhale all the air through your mouth. Continue this slow, deep breathing, in through your nose and out through your mouth, for 6 to 8 breaths.

MOVE

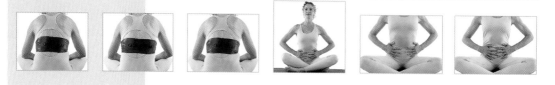

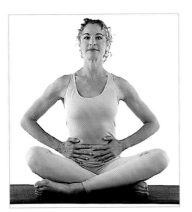

FIG. 3

FIG. 3

✳ Set your exercise band aside and sit up as tall as you can out of your hips. Place your hands on your lower abdomen with your fingers spread apart. Imagine you have a belt slung low across your hips, from headlight to headlight. Exhale all air through your mouth, imagining the belt tightening another notch.

FIG. 4

FIG. 4

✳ Count to 5 as you inhale, expanding the back and sides of your rib cage.

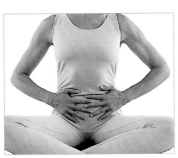

FIG. 5

FIG. 5

✳ Exhale for 5 counts, zipping vertically and tightening the belt horizontally. Your fingers should interlace across your tummy when you exhale completely. Perform 5 sets of slow, deep breathing: For each set, breathe in through your nose for 5 counts and out through your mouth for 5 counts. Then change the breathing rhythm to quick, percussive breaths and breathe in through your nose for 2 counts and out through your mouth for 2 counts. This is called the "sniff sniff, blow blow" breathing pattern. Perform 10 sets of "sniff sniff, blow blow."

OPTIONS

✳ If it's difficult for you to sit up straight in this position, take the time to place firm pillows or folded towels under your buttocks to help lengthen your spine and relax your hip joints open. If your hip joints are extremely tight, you may even want to place pillows under your knees to support them.

BODY SCAN

✳ It's not unusual to become a bit lightheaded at first during breathing practice. If you find you're straining to inhale or exhale for any reason, cut back on the length of the breath or the number of repetitions until you feel ready to do more. Advance at your own pace, and stop if you become dizzy or nauseous.

TRANSITION

✳ Remain seated for Arm Raises.

ARM RAISES

You'll integrate a simple movement into your breathing practice with Arm Raises. Lifting your arms will facilitate fully inflating your lungs. Concentrate on stabilizing your shoulders down away from your ears even as you raise your arms overhead.

BREATHE

Inhale as you raise your arms over your head, and exhale as you lower them to home position.

ENERGIZE

Visualize a marionette string extended from the crown of your head to the ceiling, and lengthen your spine up out of your hips as the string pulls upward.

ALIGN

Your shoulders should remain vertical over your hips, and your front triangles should remain overlapped as your arms rise overhead.

FIG. 1

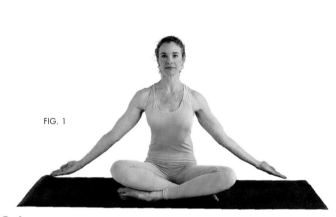

FIG. 1

✳ Sit tall with your arms stretched long at the sides of your body, palms facing up and fingertips just off the mat. Exhale all air through your mouth in home position.

MOVE

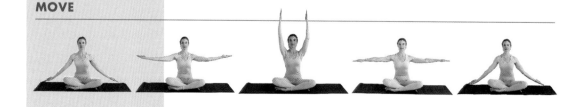

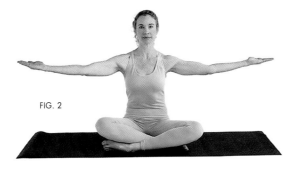

FIG. 2

✳ Begin inhaling as you raise your arms out to your sides, palms facing up.

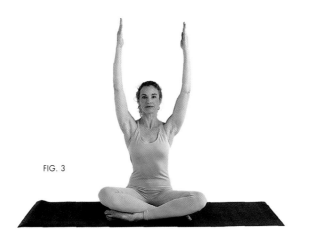

FIG. 3

✳ Finish the inhalation as your arms arrive overhead, palms facing each other. Use two-way energy. Reach up but keep your shoulders down!

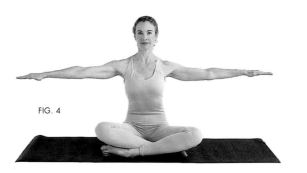

FIG. 4

✳ Rotate your palms outward, exhaling to lower your arms to home position, palms facing down. Rotate your palms up to begin again. Repeat 6 times.

OPTIONS

✳ Modify your overhead arm position to a V if you find your shoulders are lifting up.

BODY SCAN

✳ Visualize your shoulder blades sliding down into your back pockets.

✳ Avoid hunching your shoulders up around your ears as you raise your arms overhead (see page 40).

TRANSITION

✳ Come to all fours for Cat.

CAT

Pilates studied human evolution and the development of babies, and he designed many quadruped exercises. The Cat reinforces both spinal stability and mobility. Integrate the B.E.A.M. principles, paying particular attention to breath control and fluid, rhythmic movement of your spine.

BREATHE

Exhale as you round; inhale as you arch.

ENERGIZE

Feel an imaginary marionette string pulling straight out from the crown of your head, through your spine, and out your tailbone to the wall behind you.

ALIGN

Keep your knees directly under your hip joints and your hands directly under your shoulder joints at all times.

MOVE

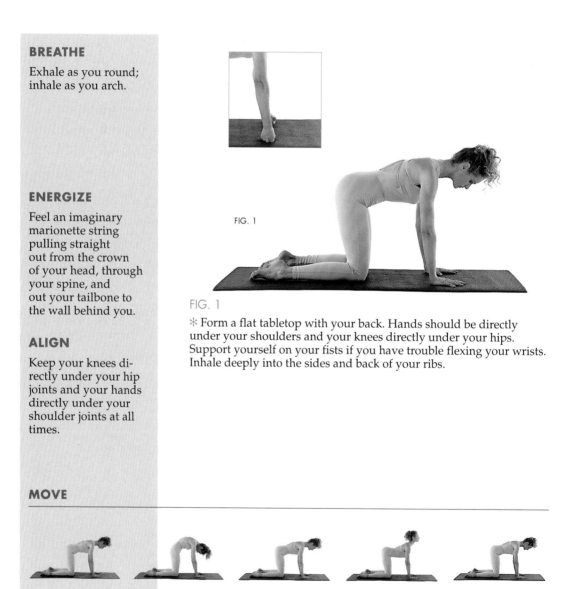

FIG. 1

FIG. 1

✳ Form a flat tabletop with your back. Hands should be directly under your shoulders and your knees directly under your hips. Support yourself on your fists if you have trouble flexing your wrists. Inhale deeply into the sides and back of your ribs.

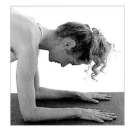

OPTIONS

❋ If you have wrist or elbow problems, support your upper body on your forearms.

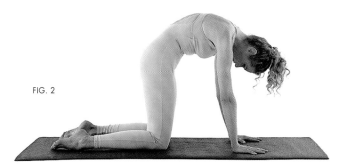

FIG. 2

FIG. 2

❋ Exhale, scooping your abs up into your spine and rounding your back like a startled cat. Pull the crown of your head and your tailbone toward one another.

BODY SCAN

❋ Avoid hunching your shoulders and locking your elbows.

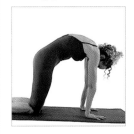

❋ Make sure not to overextend your neck.

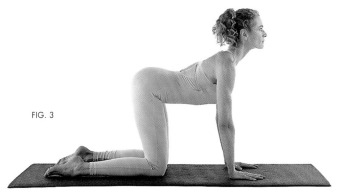

FIG. 3

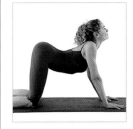

FIG. 3

❋ Inhale to reverse the curve into an arch, like the back of an old horse. No pooching abs here; stretch your front, but keep your abs scooped! Perform 4 repetitions, slowly going from cat to horse.

TRANSITION

❋ Turn onto your back, and pull your knees in to your chest for Knee Hugs.

KNEE HUGS

Knee Hugs begin a whole series of Fundamentals done lying on your back—a perfect position in which to feel your abdominals "falling into" your lower back, where they should remain when you stand up! Concentrate on maintaining a neutral pelvis and neck position here, and isolate the movement in your hip sockets.

BREATHE

Inhale in the released position; exhale when drawing your knees in.

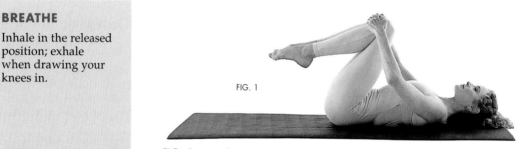

FIG. 1

FIG. 1

✳ Place a small pillow under your head and neck for the following series of exercises. Place your hands on your shins, elbows out and shoulders dropped down away from your ears. Inhale deeply through your nose in home position.

ENERGIZE

Visualize a long spine, from head to tailbone. Drop your shoulder blades down into your back pockets, and open the front of your chest.

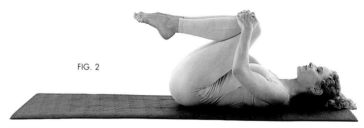

FIG. 2

ALIGN

Place a small pillow under your head and neck to help maintain the natural curve there.

FIG. 2

✳ Exhale all your air through your mouth as you hug your knees in. Inhale to release. Repeat 2 times.

MOVE

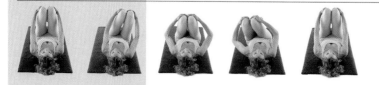

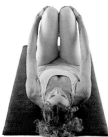

FIG. 3

FIG. 3

✳ After your final Knee Hug, inhale in home position.

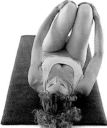

FIG. 4

FIG. 4

✳ Begin exhaling as you draw both knees toward your right armpit.

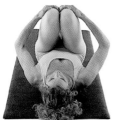

FIG. 5

FIG. 5

✳ Continue exhaling as you draw both knees across the center of your chest.

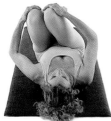

FIG. 6

FIG. 6

✳ Finish the exhale as you draw both knees toward your left armpit.

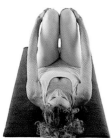

FIG. 7

FIG. 7

✳ Inhale as you return to home position. Perform 3 circles, exhaling with each circular pull across your chest. Then perform 3 circles in the opposite direction.

OPTIONS

✳ If you have a knee problem, you can place your hands behind your knees.

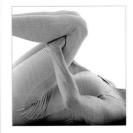

BODY SCAN

✳ Draw your knees toward your chest, not your shoulders toward your knees!

✳ Keep your neck in a neutral position. Avoid tilting your head back.

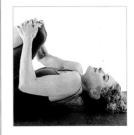

TRANSITION

✳ Keep your right knee bent and extend your left leg long on the mat for Knee Stirs.

KNEE STIRS

Knee Stirs isolate the circular movement of the thighbone in the hip socket. These exercises also develop awareness of the need to balance flexibility in the hip with stability in the pelvis, which should remain anchored throughout the exercise. Keep the stirs small, and exhale to accent the ab scoop as you return to home position.

BREATHE

Inhale as you begin the circle; exhale to complete it.

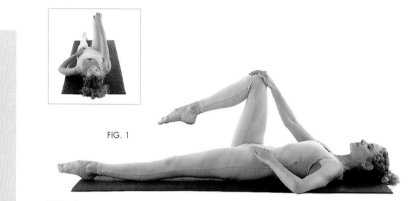

FIG. 1

ENERGIZE

Imagine your hip socket is a mortar and your thighbone is a lightly stirring pestle.

FIG. 1

❋ Place your left hand on your left headlight, and hold your right kneecap lightly with your right hand.

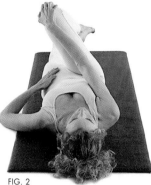

FIG. 2

ALIGN

Stabilize your pelvis by engaging all the muscles in your Powerhouse. Align your supporting leg directly under your hip, as if you were standing on one leg.

FIG. 2

FIG. 2

❋ Inhale as you lightly "stir" your right thigh across your body toward your left armpit.

MOVE

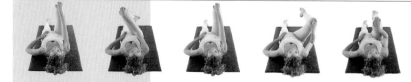

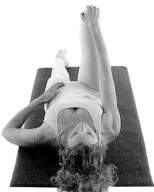

FIG. 3

FIG. 3

✳ Continue stirring your knee down and away through the midline of your body.

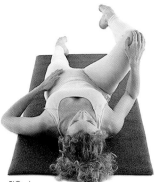

FIG. 4

FIG. 4

✳ Begin exhaling as you open your knee toward the armpit. Keep your left headlight anchored!

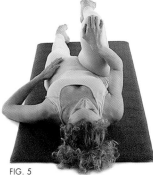

FIG. 5

FIG. 5

✳ Finish as you circle your knee across your chest. Perform 3 stirs in each direction. To change legs, inhale deeply. On the next exhalation, draw your left knee in to your chest and stretch your right leg out onto the floor. Place your right hand on your right headlight. Hold your left kneecap lightly with your left hand. Perform 3 stirs in each direction.

OPTIONS

✳ If your lower back or legs feel strained with your supporting leg fully extended on the floor, bend your supporting leg and place your foot flat on the mat.

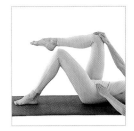

BODY SCAN

✳ Avoid tilting your headlights from side to side as you stir the knee.

✳ Isolate the movement in your hip socket and keep your headlights balanced.

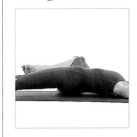

TRANSITION

✳ Bend both knees, feet on the mat, directly in line with your hip sockets for Pelvic Tuck and Arch.

PELVIC TUCK AND ARCH

This exercise helps you identify your own neutral pelvis position while lying on your back and gives you practice in actively scooping your lower abs without engaging your buttocks muscles. Keep the movements small, precise, and well coordinated with your breath. (*Note:* You've already practiced this skill in vertical alignment in Chapter 2; see page 36.)

BREATHE

Exhale to tuck your pelvis; inhale to arch.

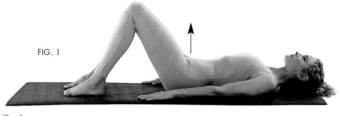

FIG. 1

FIG. 1

✳ Lie on your back in neutral spine with your knees bent, feet hip-width apart, and arms stretched long at your sides. (*Note:* Your arms remain in this position throughout the exercise. Later photos show the arm moved only to reveal the pelvic movement.) Inhale through your nose to the sides and back of your ribs.

ENERGIZE

Visualize a long, flexible spine from head to tailbone, and see your headlights shining directly on the ceiling in the starting position.

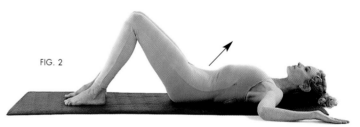

FIG. 2

FIG. 2

✳ Exhale. Scoop out your lower abs to flatten the small of your back into the mat for the Pelvic Tuck. The pubic bone tilts up in this position, and your headlights point up toward your chin. Isolate your deepest lower abdominal muscles to flatten your spine, with no help from your buttocks muscles.

ALIGN

Stretch your arms down alongside your body, palms pressed into the mat. Draw your shoulders down away from your ears. Feel the tripod of each foot rooted firmly into the mat.

MOVE

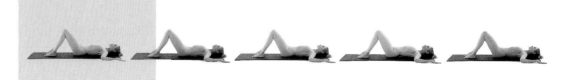

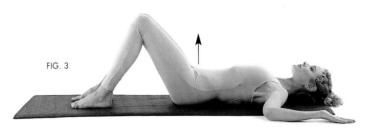

FIG. 3

FIG. 3

✳ Inhale. Return to neutral. Exhale, holding neutral without changing your alignment.

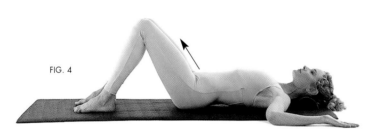

FIG. 4

FIG. 4

✳ Inhale. Overarch your lower back. The space between your lower back and the mat enlarges slightly. Your pubic bone tilts down, and your headlights shine toward your bent knees. Note the enlarged space between the lower back and the mat in the arched position.

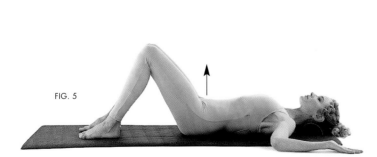

FIG. 5

FIG. 5

✳ Exhale to return to neutral. Repeat once slowly; then move faster, tucking and arching for 4 repetitions without stopping in neutral.

OPTIONS

✳ As you progress, move your feet farther away from your buttocks for a greater challenge.

BODY SCAN

✳ *Don't* tense your buttocks or lower back muscles. Isolate your deepest lower abdominal muscles to flatten your spine without pooching your belly.

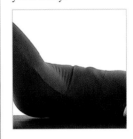

✳ Keep the arch small and confined to your lower back. Do not arch in your middle or upper back.

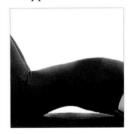

TRANSITION

✳ Remove the pillow from behind your head for Chin Tuck and Neck Arch.

CHIN TUCK AND NECK ARCH

These exercises help identify a neutral position for your head, neck, and shoulders, so your head is carried on the top of your spine in a relaxed, efficient position.

BREATHE

Exhale to tuck or arch; inhale to return to neutral.

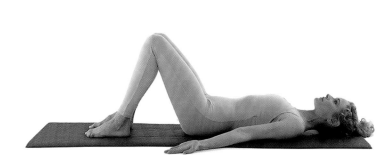

ENERGIZE

Imagine a marionette string extending upward from the crown of your head, lengthening your neck.

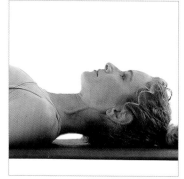

FIG. 1

ALIGN

Your head is in neutral when your jawbone forms a right angle to your neck. As in neutral pelvis, there will be some air space between your neck and the mat.

FIG. 1

※ Inhale in the neutral spine position with your knees bent, feet flat on the mat, arms reaching down along your sides, palms facing up.

MOVE

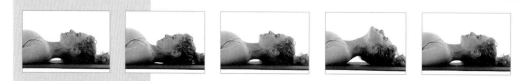

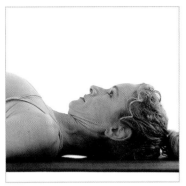

FIG. 2

FIG. 2

✳ Exhale; tuck your chin down toward your chest, and lengthen the back of your neck into the mat.

OPTIONS

✳ If your shoulders are tense, widen your arms away from your body and turn your palms up.

BODY SCAN

✳ Avoid an extreme overarch of your neck, which can compress the cervical vertebrae.

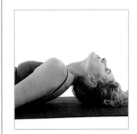

✳ Keep your shoulders drawn down away from your ears at all times.

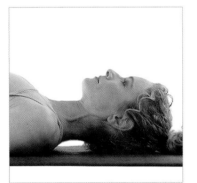

FIG. 3

FIG. 3

✳ Inhale as you relax and return to neutral.

TRANSITION

✳ Move your mat near a wall for Pistons, and replace the pillow to support your head and neck.

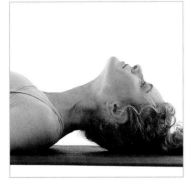

FIG. 4

FIG. 4

✳ Exhale. Overarch your neck, looking upside-down at the wall behind you. Inhale as you return to neutral. Perform 4 slow repetitions, stopping in neutral. Then perform 8 quick repetitions, exhaling to tuck and inhaling to arch.

PISTONS

The Pistons challenge you to stabilize your body in neutral while moving your legs. This exercise looks easy, but when it's done properly, you should feel your lower abdominal muscles working hard to maintain a neutral spine as you move your legs.

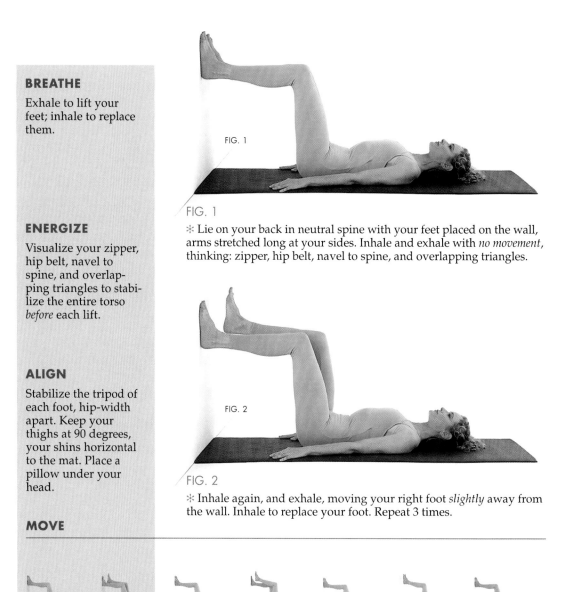

BREATHE

Exhale to lift your feet; inhale to replace them.

FIG. 1

FIG. 1

✳ Lie on your back in neutral spine with your feet placed on the wall, arms stretched long at your sides. Inhale and exhale with *no movement*, thinking: zipper, hip belt, navel to spine, and overlapping triangles.

ENERGIZE

Visualize your zipper, hip belt, navel to spine, and overlapping triangles to stabilize the entire torso *before* each lift.

ALIGN

Stabilize the tripod of each foot, hip-width apart. Keep your thighs at 90 degrees, your shins horizontal to the mat. Place a pillow under your head.

FIG. 2

FIG. 2

✳ Inhale again, and exhale, moving your right foot *slightly* away from the wall. Inhale to replace your foot. Repeat 3 times.

MOVE

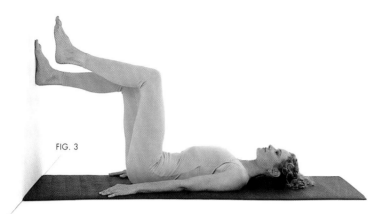

FIG. 3

✳ Inhale and exhale again with no movement, to stabilize. Inhale, and then exhale to move your left foot *slightly* away from the wall. Inhale to replace your foot. Repeat 3 times.

✳ Now make it a bit more challenging: Inhale and exhale with no movement to stabilize. Inhale and exhale, removing your *right* foot, and hold it in the air. Inhale here, exhale, and remove your *left* foot. Inhale, holding both legs up. Exhale; replace the *right* foot. Inhale, hold, and exhale to replace the *left* foot.

✳ Next, reverse the pattern: Inhale with no movement and exhale to remove the *left* foot; hold it in the air. Inhale here, and then exhale to remove the *right* foot. Inhale, holding both legs up. Exhale; replace the *left*. Inhale, hold, then exhale to replace the *right* foot. Perform 3 sets.

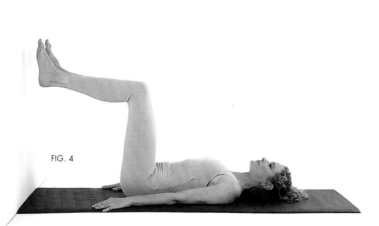

FIG. 4

✳ Inhale and exhale with no movement, thinking: zipper, hip belt, navel to spine, and overlapping triangles. Inhale again, and exhale to remove both feet simultaneously, keeping your spine neutral and your abs scooped. Inhale to replace your feet. Repeat 3 times.

OPTIONS

✳ For more of a challenge, work up to performing Pistons with your feet on the floor.

BODY SCAN

✳ Keep your arms stretched long at your sides. Draw your shoulders down away from your ears. Relax your neck and jaw.

✳ Be sure not to pooch your abs out as you exhale.

TRANSITION

✳ Remain lying on your back with your feet hip-width apart on the wall for Pelvic Press, and remove your neck pillow.

PELVIC PRESS

This is a wonderful exercise to teach two key Pilates concepts: spinal articulation and imprinting. Focus on isolating each vertebra as you peel your spine off the mat, and imprint one vertebra at a time as you roll back down.

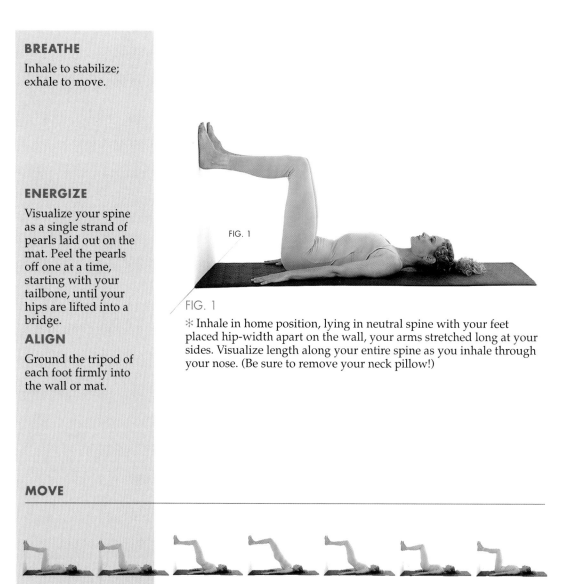

FIG. 1

FIG. 1

✳ Inhale in home position, lying in neutral spine with your feet placed hip-width apart on the wall, your arms stretched long at your sides. Visualize length along your entire spine as you inhale through your nose. (Be sure to remove your neck pillow!)

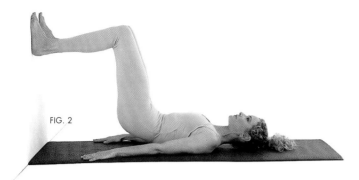

FIG. 2

* Move through Pelvic Tuck as you exhale. This time, *do* engage your buttocks as you roll up into a full Pelvic Press.

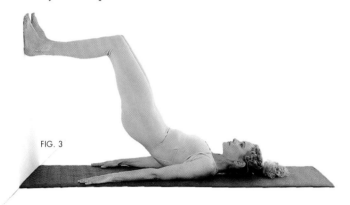

FIG. 3

* Articulate each vertebra individually, as you peel off the mat.

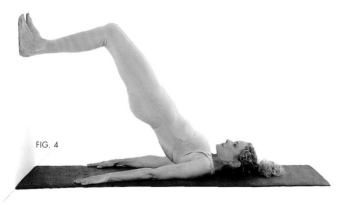

FIG. 4

* Inhale when you reach the top of your Pelvic Press, then exhale to roll down, imprinting each vertebra into the mat to return to home position. Repeat 4 times. Hug your knees in to your chest to rest for a moment.

OPTIONS

* For more of a challenge, work up to performing Pelvic Press starting with your feet on the floor.

BODY SCAN

* Avoid popping the triangles apart in front of your body.

* Avoid overarching your back. If you feel any lower back pressure, you've rolled up too high and your smile muscles are likely not engaged.

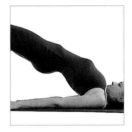

TRANSITION

* If you've had your feet on the wall, move back to the center of your mat for Cross-Leg Fall, and replace the pillow under your head and neck.

CROSS-LEG FALL

Cross-Leg Fall is a great way to work your oblique abdominals without straining your neck and shoulders. It will help trim your waist and reinforce spinal imprinting on a diagonal.

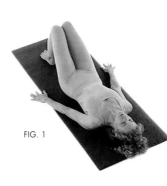

FIG. 1

BREATHE

Inhale with no movement; move on the exhalation.

FIG. 1

✳ Inhale and exhale deeply to stabilize your center in home position.

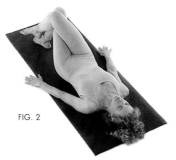

FIG. 2

ENERGIZE

Visualize a highway line down the center of your mat. Start on the line, fall to the side, and imprint back onto it.

FIG. 2

✳ Lift your right leg and cross your thighs, right over left. Inhale again, holding the cross-leg position.

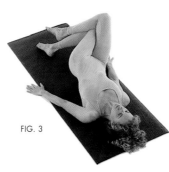

FIG. 3

ALIGN

Lie on your back in neutral with your knees bent, and place a pillow under your head or neck. Press your knees and feet together, and stretch your arms long at the sides of your body.

FIG. 3

✳ Exhale, allowing both legs to fall right. Keep both shoulders squarely on the mat and your head in neutral. Inhale, *holding* the position. Begin exhaling as you slowly draw the left side of your ribs to the mat. Imprint the upper spine, navel to spine, hip belt, and zipper as you finish the exhale to return home.

MOVE

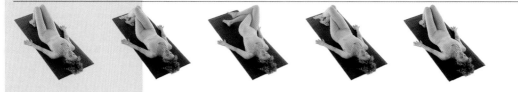

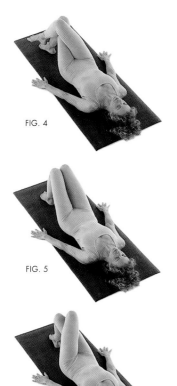

FIG. 4

FIG. 4

✳ Inhale in home position with your right leg crossed over left. Exhale; fall again to the right. Repeat 3 times.

FIG. 5

✳ Unhook your right leg, and replace it on the mat.

FIG. 5

FIG. 6

✳ Inhale and exhale deeply to stabilize your center as you lift your left leg and cross your thighs, left over right. Inhale again, holding the cross-leg position.

FIG. 6

FIG. 7

✳ Exhale, allowing *both* legs to fall left. Keep both shoulders squarely on the mat and your head in neutral. Inhale, holding the position.

FIG. 7

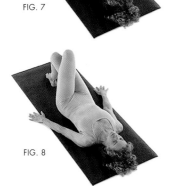

FIG. 8

✳ Begin exhaling as you slowly draw the right side of your ribs to the mat. Imprint your upper spine, navel to spine, hip belt, and zipper as you finish the exhale to return home. Inhale in home position, left leg crossed over right. Exhale; fall again to the left. Repeat 3 times.

FIG. 8

OPTIONS

✳ Hold small hand-balls or tennis balls in both hands. As you exhale to return to neutral, squeeze the ball on the active side to stabilize your shoulder down and engage your obliques.

BODY SCAN

✳ Keep your upper body and head in neutral position throughout the entire exercise.

✳ Don't initiate your return to home position with hips or buttocks muscles! Keep them relaxed and use your abs to imprint your spine.

TRANSITION

✳ Unhook your left leg, and replace your foot on the mat. Bend your knees, and place your feet hip-width apart to prepare for Puppet Arms.

PUPPET ARMS

Puppet Arms is more of a releasing than a strengthening exercise. Using the force of gravity, you will learn to drop your shoulders away from your ears and train your shoulder blades to lie flat against the back of your ribs. Once your upper body is correctly placed, you can begin the strengthening exercises.

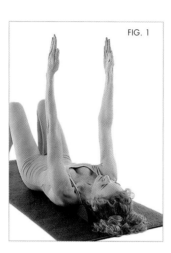

FIG. 1

BREATHE

Inhale to stretch away from the mat, and exhale to drop your arms.

FIG. 1

✳ Lie on your back in neutral spine with knees bent, hip-width apart. Raise both arms into the air in a direct vertical line over your shoulders. The palms of your hands should face one another. Exhale to empty your lungs completely in home position.

ENERGIZE

Imagine your fingers are suspended from the ceiling by marionette strings. The strings will alternately pull and release.

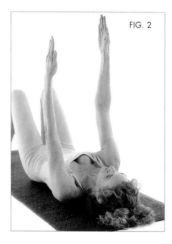

FIG. 2

ALIGN

Be sure your arms are at a 90-degree angle to your torso. Maintain a neutral spine throughout the exercise.

FIG. 2

✳ Inhale. Raise the back of your right shoulder off the floor, reaching your fingertips toward the ceiling.

MOVE

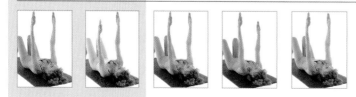

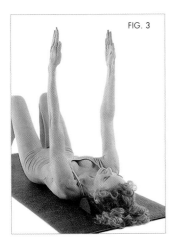

FIG. 3

✳ Exhale. Drop your shoulder back to the mat.

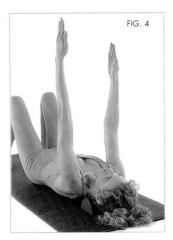

FIG. 4

✳ Inhale. Raise the back of your left shoulder off the floor, reaching your fingertips toward the ceiling.

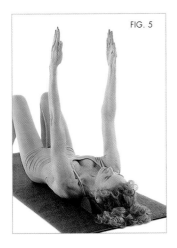

FIG. 5

✳ Exhale. Drop your shoulder back to the mat. Perform 3 repetitions lifting each arm separately; then perform 3 repetitions lifting both arms together.

OPTIONS

✳ Hold 1-to-2-pound hand weights.

BODY SCAN

✳ Lift your shoulders toward the ceiling, *not* toward your ears. Keep your neck relaxed.

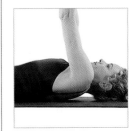

TRANSITION

✳ Turn the palms of your hands to face down toward your feet for Arm Circles.

ARM CIRCLES

Arm Circles help to open tight shoulders and upper back muscles as you work to keep your upper torso stabilized. Limit the size of your circles at first, and let gravity help to move your arms freely from your shoulders.

FIG. 1

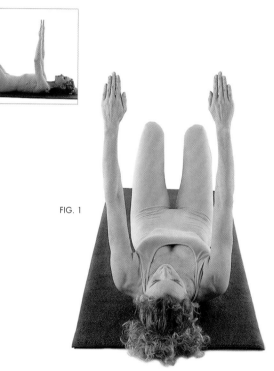

FIG. 1

BREATHE

Inhale as your arms circle away from you; exhale as they close.

ENERGIZE

Keep the points of the front triangles overlapping throughout this exercise. Imagine your fingertips tracing the inside of a large bubble.

ALIGN

Be sure your hands are in a direct vertical line over your shoulders, and your palms are facing your feet.

FIG. 1

⁕ Home position is identical to Puppet Arms, but your palms face down toward your feet to begin. Inhale and then exhale in home position to ground your center.

MOVE

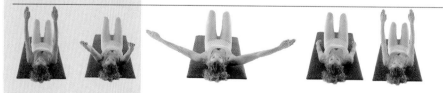

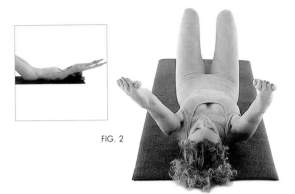

FIG. 2

FIG. 2

✳ Inhale as your hands reach back overhead. Keep the front of your ribs pressed down—triangles remain overlapping.

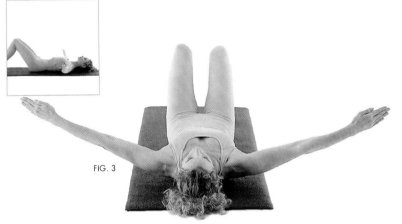

FIG. 3

FIG. 3

✳ Begin to exhale, opening your arms to the sides.

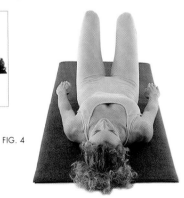

FIG. 4

FIG. 4

✳ Finish the exhalation as you complete the Arm Circle, bringing your hands close to your hips, palms facing down. Do 3 circles in each direction.

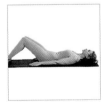

OPTIONS

✳ Hold 1-to-2-pound hand weights.

BODY SCAN

✳ Draw your shoulders down away from your ears as your arms circle. Avoid letting the triangles on the front of your body separate when your arms are in the overhead position.

TRANSITION

✳ Remove your pillow and turn onto your stomach for V-Pull and Elbow Push-Up.

V-PULL AND ELBOW PUSH-UP

V-Pull is a fabulous exercise for your pelvic floor, abs, buttocks, and inner thighs. Here you'll work your abs against gravity—which is more challenging than when lying on your back. Elbow Push-Up is for folks who have winged or protruding shoulder blades when in a push-up or all-fours position. It's also good for those who have flattened their thoracic curve. It strengthens the muscles that hold the shoulder blades close to the ribs. Do these exercises before more advanced work, such as push-ups or Airplane.

BREATHE

Inhale in the home position; exhale to form the tunnel under your waistline (see Fig. 2). Inhale in the home position, and exhale to push up (see Fig. 4).

ENERGIZE

Feel that you could drive a toy car under your navel during the exhale (see Fig. 2). Form a tripod with your forearms. Drive your elbows into the mat as you push up (see Fig. 4).

ALIGN

The natural curve of your lower back flattens as you tuck your pelvis (see Fig. 2).

Position your elbows so they come in to line with your shoulders when you push up (see Fig. 4).

MOVE

FIG. 1

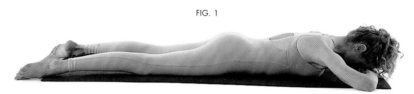

FIG. 1
✳ Lie facedown on the mat with your hands stacked under your forehead and your legs slightly apart. Inhale.

FIG. 2

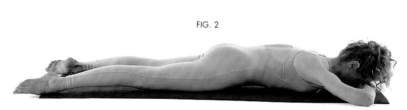

FIG. 2
✳ Exhale to tuck your pelvis, lift your abs, and engage your Powerhouse to form a tunnel under your waistline. Hold for 4 counts. Inhale to release. Repeat 3 to 5 times total.

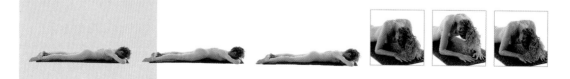

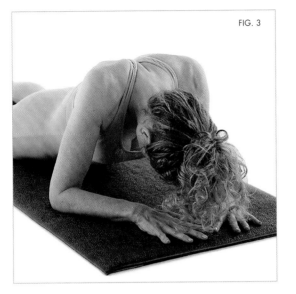

FIG. 3

FIG. 3

* Inhale, allowing the top of your head to drop toward the mat.

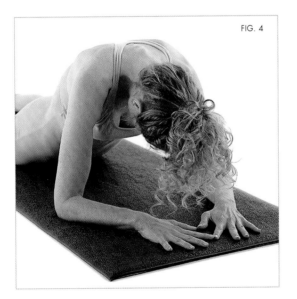

FIG. 4

FIG. 4

* Exhale to push up, pulling your chin to your chest and stretching your shoulder blades apart. Hold for 4 counts. Release as you inhale. Repeat 3 to 5 times total.

OPTIONS

* If your lower back is tight, place a pillow under your hips for V-Pull (see photo on page 79).

* If Elbow Push-Up on the mat is too difficult, lean against a wall.

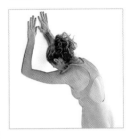

BODY SCAN

* Avoid lifting your buttocks to form the tunnel. Press your pubic bone firmly into the mat.

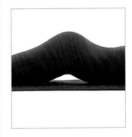

TRANSITION

* Remain on your stomach for Back Extensions, or skip ahead to page 80 for Airplane.

BACK EXTENSIONS

This series helps strengthen your back and the muscles that keep your shoulders down. It has four phases and can be performed either with your head resting on a pillow or your upper body hovering off the mat. Take time learning each phase, because each movement builds on the previous one. The initial phases are very beneficial; move on only when you have mastered the basics.

BREATHE

Inhale to prepare and stabilize your shoulders down, and exhale to move.

ENERGIZE

Visualize two-way energy: a marionette string out of the top of your head and shoulder blades drawn down into your back pockets.

ALIGN

In the prone position, a pillow under your forehead will help to keep your neck in neutral alignment and help you avoid smashing your nose.

MOVE

FIG. 1

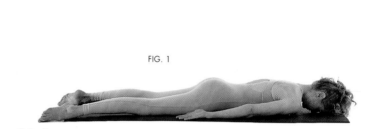

FIG. 1

✳ Place your forehead on the mat and stretch your arms down long at your sides, palms facing *up*. Inhale in home position.

FIG. 2

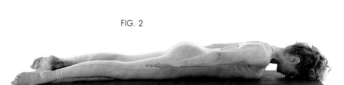

FIG. 2

✳ Exhale to lengthen your fingertips to your ankles. Draw your shoulder blades down into your back pockets, and lift your arms to hover slightly off the mat. Inhale to release to home position. Repeat.

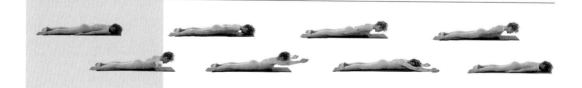

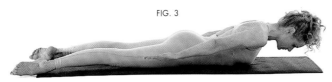

FIG. 3

FIG. 3

✳ Inhale in home position (see Fig. 1). Exhale, engage your Powerhouse, and lengthen to lift your entire upper body to hover off the mat. Keep the back of your neck long. Inhale to release to home position. Repeat.

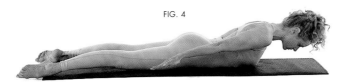

FIG. 4

FIG. 4

✳ Inhale in home position. Exhale, engage your Powerhouse, and lengthen to lift your entire upper body to hover off the mat (see Fig. 3). Inhale and *hold* the position, but rotate the palms of your hands *down*.

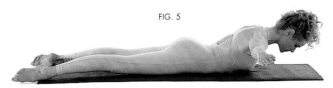

FIG. 5

FIG. 5

✳ Exhale, and *slowly* reach your arms out to your sides at shoulder height, palms facing *down*. *Lengthen* to come down to the mat. Inhale and return to home position, palms facing *up*. Repeat Steps 4 and 5.

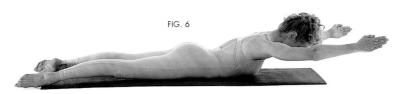

FIG. 6

FIG. 6

✳ Inhale in home position. Exhale, engage your Powerhouse, and lengthen to lift and hover your entire upper body off the mat (see Fig. 3). Inhale and *hold* the position, but rotate the palms of your hands *down* (see Fig. 4). Exhale, and *slowly* reach your arms out to your sides (see Fig. 5). Inhale and *hold* this position, but rotate your palms forward. Exhale to bring your arms to a V position, framing your head. Keep your shoulders down! *Lengthen* to come down to the mat. Inhale and return to home position, palms facing up. Repeat.

OPTIONS

✳ If your neck strains easily, rest your forehead on a pillow and perform only the arm movements.

✳ If your lower back is tight, place a pillow under your hips.

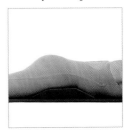

BODY SCAN

✳ Avoid overextending your neck and hunching your shoulders.

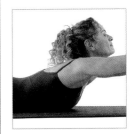

TRANSITION

✳ Remain in home position (see Fig. 1).

To move into Rest Position, skip to page 82.

AIRPLANE

This is a good exercise if you're uncomfortable lying on your stomach, as in Back Extensions. Airplane is excellent for strengthening all the muscles on the back of your body: back extensors, buttocks, and hamstrings. At the same time, your abdominals and shoulder stabilizers must work to keep your pelvis and hips level throughout.

BREATHE

Exhale as you lift your arm and leg.

ENERGIZE

Visualize a long line of energy from the tips of your fingers to the tips of your toes in the extended position.

ALIGN

Maintain neutral shoulders and hips throughout the exercise.

MOVE

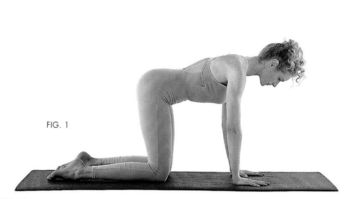

FIG. 1

FIG. 1

✳ Form a flat tabletop with your back. Align your knees directly under your hip joints and your hands directly under your shoulder joints. Inhale and exhale to ground yourself in home position. Inhale once again.

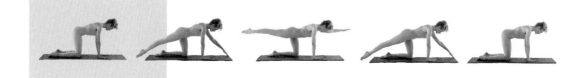

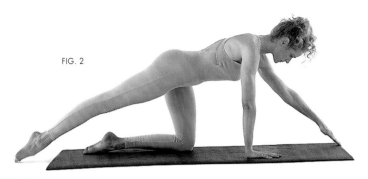

FIG. 2

FIG. 2

* As you exhale, extend your opposite hand and leg along the mat as far as they can reach while maintaining contact with the floor. Use your Powerhouse to keep your hips stable, and stabilize your shoulder blades down into your back pockets to avoid hunching. Inhale while *holding* this position.

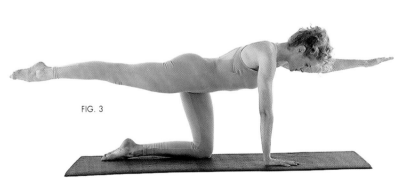
FIG. 3

FIG. 3

* Exhale to lift your arm and leg to horizontal. Inhale to touch down; exhale to lift off to horizontal again. Touch down and lift off 3 times. Return to home position, and switch sides to perform 3 more repetitions.

OPTIONS

* If you find your shoulders hunching, don't lift your arm fully to horizontal. Lift only as high as you can while stabilizing your shoulders down.

BODY SCAN

* Keep your head-lights and shoulders level at all times.

* Lifting your working leg too high will cause your lower back to overarch.

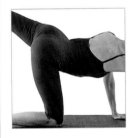

* Shoulder blades should rest flat against your rib cage.

* Keep the line of your extended arm, leg, and torso parallel to your mat.

TRANSITION

* Sit your buttocks back toward your heels as you move into Rest Position.

REST POSITION

Rest Position is restorative. It's a great place to practice deep lateral breathing into the sides and back of your ribs. Additionally, you'll stretch out your lower back, shoulders, and neck. Move into Rest Position anytime you feel the need during your workout.

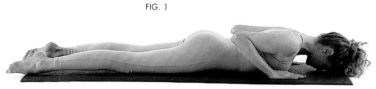

FIG. 1

BREATHE

Stay in Rest Position for several cycles of deep breathing.

FIG. 1

 From the prone position, place your hands, palms down, directly under your shoulder joints, elbows in.

ENERGIZE

Inflate your ribs horizontally, like an accordion, as you inhale. As you exhale, activate your zipper, hip belt, and navel to spine to engage your lower abs.

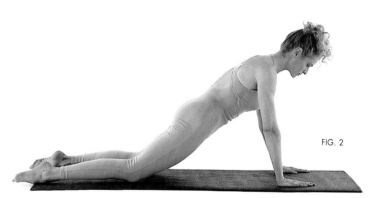

FIG. 2

ALIGN

Place your knees hip-width apart and your hands shoulder-width apart.

FIG. 2

 Straighten your arms, lifting your upper body.

MOVE

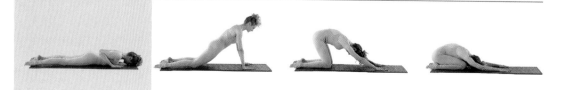

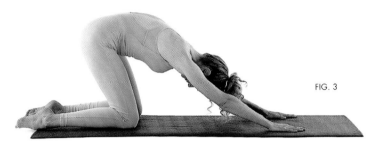

FIG. 3

FIG. 3

* Exhale as you round your back, drop your head, engage your abdominals, and sit your buttocks toward your heels.

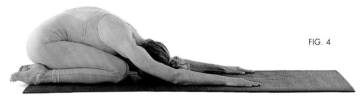

FIG. 4

FIG. 4

* In Rest Position, relax your forehead to the mat and your buttocks toward your heels. Stretch your arms long overhead, palms down. Continue breathing deeply. Scoop out your lower abs as you exhale, thinking: zipper, hip belt, navel to spine. Roll your forehead from side to side, as if you're shaking your head "no." Release any tight muscles in your neck and shoulders. Allow your buttocks to become heavier, sinking farther toward your heels with each exhale.

OPTIONS

* Stretch your arms alongside your body, palms up. As needed, place pillows under your forehead, stomach, buttocks, and feet for support.

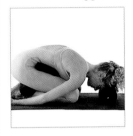

* Stack your fists under your forehead.

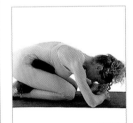

BODY SCAN

* Fully inflate and deflate your lungs.

* Relax your neck and shoulders as you inhale.

TRANSITION

* Turn onto your back and place a pillow under your head and neck for Foot Flex/Point and Ankle Circles.

FOOT FLEX/POINT AND ANKLE CIRCLES

The feet and ankles are the foundation of your vertical posture and are too often ignored when working out. These exercises will strengthen the muscles of your feet and ankles and train you to maintain proper knee, ankle, and foot alignment.

BREATHE

Inhale to flex, and exhale to point.

Inhale as you begin the circle and exhale to return home.

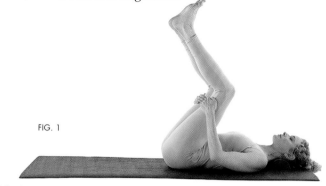

FIG. 1

ENERGIZE

Articulate your feet as if they were hands. Extend energy through all five toes.

Keep energy reaching through your toes to create the largest circle possible.

ALIGN

Form a straight line from the center of each hip joint through the knee joint and out through the center of each foot, running between the second and third toes in the home position.

MOVE

FIG. 1

❋ Lie on your back with both legs raised, hip-width apart, with knees bent. Hold the back of your thighs for support. Inhale, then exhale with your feet relaxed in home position.

FIG. 2

❋ Begin inhaling as you make "fists" with your feet, grasping your toes together into a ball.

FIG. 3

❋ Open your toes and flex your forefeet back, reaching through your heels.

FIG. 4

❋ Begin to exhale as you point your feet, reaching through the heels and balls of your feet.

FIG. 5

❋ Complete the exhale as you finish the point, without clenching your toes. Flex back through your toes, balls of your feet, and heels. Inhale to make fists again. Repeat 4 times.

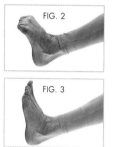

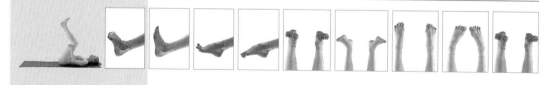

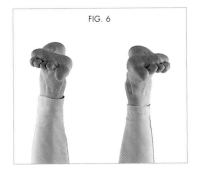

FIG. 6

❊ When you've completed the last flex/point, relax in home position with hips, knees, ankles, and feet in good parallel alignment. Then flex your feet again, toes pulled back, reaching through your heels.

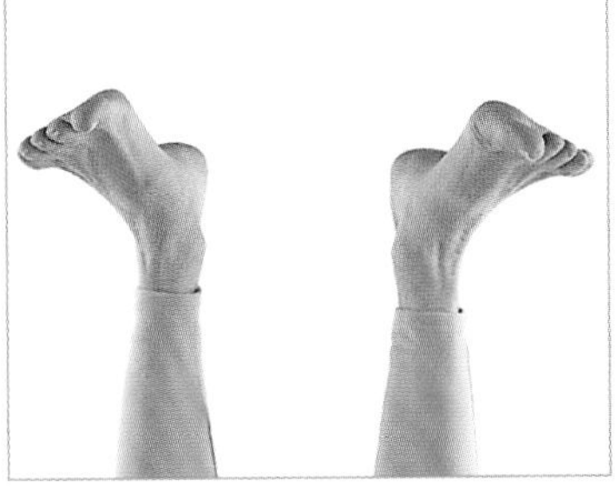

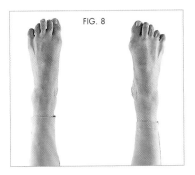

FIG. 7

❊ Inhale as you begin circling your feet around to the outside.

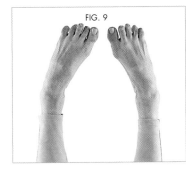

FIG. 8

❊ Reach to a full point without gripping your toes.

FIG. 9

❊ Exhale as your feet circle inward and flex back to the parallel flex position (see Fig. 6).

❊ Pause for a moment in good alignment as you complete each circle, training yourself to automatically use your foot correctly.

❊ Do 4 circles one way; then reverse and do 4 the other way.

BODY SCAN

❊ Isolate the movement in your feet and ankles only, keeping your hips and knees quiet.

❊ Be sure to perform complete circles in each direction.

TRANSITION

❊ When you've completed the last circle, place one foot down on the mat for Hamstring Stretch.

HAMSTRING STRETCH

You need flexible hamstrings in order to correctly perform many of the classic Pilates exercises. This stretch series will teach you to isolate this important muscle group and open up the backs of your legs. Stretching will help you avoid injury and prepare you for the more rigorous exercises to come.

BREATHE

Inhale to back off the stretch; exhale to deepen it.

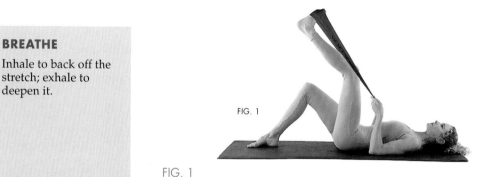

FIG. 1

FIG. 1

ENERGIZE

Visualize two-way energy: Pull your navel to spine and reach your leg out as far as possible.

※ Lie on your back in neutral spine with one foot flat on the mat, knee bent. Place an exercise band around the sole of the other foot and extend your leg in the air, slightly bent. Inhale in home position.

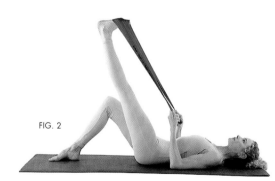

FIG. 2

ALIGN

Maintain good horizontal shoulder and hip alignment throughout the exercise, and remember to maintain a neutral spine. Tucking your pelvis creates the illusion of more flexible hamstrings.

FIG. 2

※ Exhale, activating your Powerhouse to straighten your knee. Repeat 3 times, and hold the last one straight. Inhale once again.

MOVE

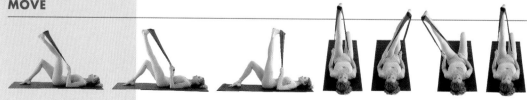

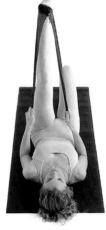

FIG. 3

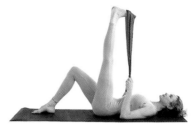

FIG. 3

✳ Exhale to gently stretch your leg toward your chest. Inhale to back off the stretch; exhale to deepen. Repeat 3 times, keeping your leg in line with your hip socket.

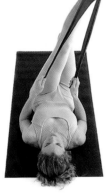

FIG. 4

FIG. 4

✳ Release the stretch and bring your leg slightly across your body, toward your opposite shoulder. This stretch is more difficult, so don't overdo it! Inhale to release; exhale to stretch diagonally. Repeat 3 times.

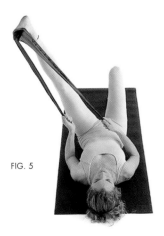

FIG. 5

FIG. 5

✳ Release, and open your leg slightly toward your other shoulder now, keeping the opposite side of your pelvis level. Inhale to release; exhale to stretch. Repeat 3 times and then change legs. Be sure to begin in home position (see Fig. 1) for the other leg.

OPTIONS

✳ As you become more flexible, try these exercises with your supporting leg straight against the mat.

BODY SCAN

✳ Avoid tucking your pelvis or lifting your lower back off the mat.

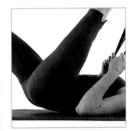

✳ Keep your supporting leg in alignment under your hip.

TRANSITION

✳ Bend both knees in to your chest, and put your exercise band aside. Come back to a neutral spine with both feet flat on the mat and your knees bent for Head Float and Rib Slide.

HEAD FLOAT AND RIB SLIDE

These two exercises are a breakdown of the traditional abdominal crunch. Unlike crunches, they should be performed in *slow motion*. Focus on the support of your lower abs to prevent abdominal pooching, and visualize overlapping the triangles on the front of your torso to raise your upper body off the mat.

BREATHE

Inhale in home position; exhale to lift.

FIG. 1

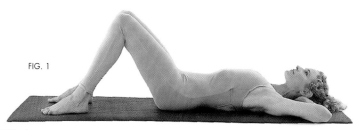

FIG. 1

✳ Interlace your hands at the base of your skull with your elbows out. Focus your eyes directly above you on the ceiling, keeping your neck relaxed. Inhale in home position.

ENERGIZE

Make your head heavy in your hands for Head Float, as if holding a bowling ball.

For Rib Slide, visualize your lowest ribs sliding down toward your hipbones.

ALIGN

Maintain neutral neck alignment and a neutral spine throughout the movement.

FIG. 2

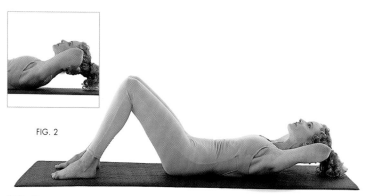

FIG. 2

✳ Exhale, activating your zipper, hip belt, navel to spine, and triangles as you raise your upper body *slightly* off the mat. Keep your head heavy in your hands. Look straight at the ceiling, and maintain a neutral spine. Inhale to return to home position. Repeat 5 to 10 times. After the final repetition, hold the Head Float and move to Rib Slide.

MOVE

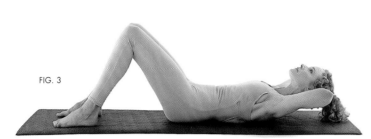

FIG. 3

FIG. 3

* To begin the Rib Slide, hold the last Head Float up. Inhale.

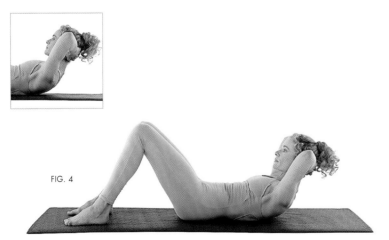

FIG. 4

FIG. 4

* Exhale, activating your zipper, hip belt, and navel to spine, to raise your upper body higher, overlapping your triangles even closer together. Focus your eyes on your kneecaps. Inhale to release back to Head Float. Repeat 5 to 10 times; then relax your upper body back to the mat (see Fig. 1).

OPTIONS

* If you experience tension in your neck, use a hand towel under your upper back and head to provide support. Relax the back of your skull into the towel as if your head were hanging in a hammock.

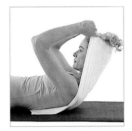

BODY SCAN

* Avoid initiating the movement with your head, neck, or shoulders.

* Keep the back of your neck lengthened and avoid over-arching.

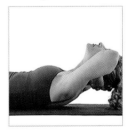

TRANSITION

* Draw one leg at a time into the air to prepare for Mini Breathing. Use your Powerhouse and don't pooch.

MINI BREATHING

This is our first classic Pilates exercise, the Breathing 100s, albeit in a supermodified form. Here we merge the controlled percussive and long breathing from our Seated Breathing practice into the intense abdominal work Pilates is famous for.

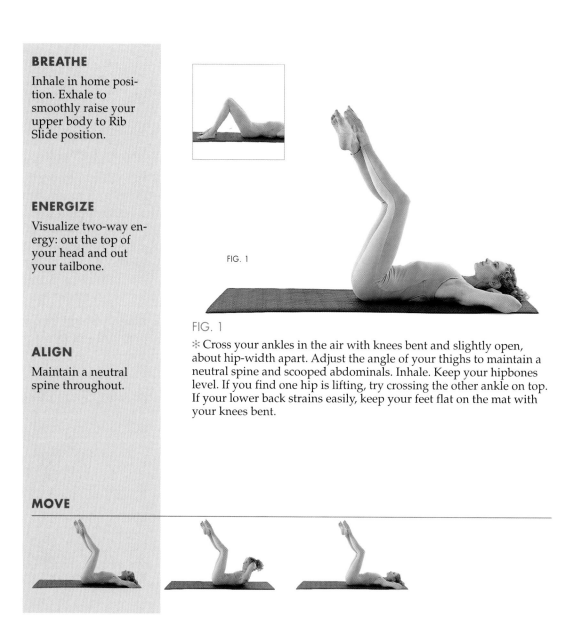

BREATHE

Inhale in home position. Exhale to smoothly raise your upper body to Rib Slide position.

ENERGIZE

Visualize two-way energy: out the top of your head and out your tailbone.

FIG. 1

ALIGN

Maintain a neutral spine throughout.

FIG. 1

✳ Cross your ankles in the air with knees bent and slightly open, about hip-width apart. Adjust the angle of your thighs to maintain a neutral spine and scooped abdominals. Inhale. Keep your hipbones level. If you find one hip is lifting, try crossing the other ankle on top. If your lower back strains easily, keep your feet flat on the mat with your knees bent.

MOVE

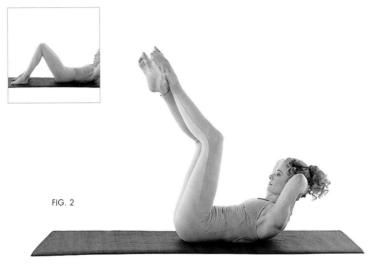

FIG. 2

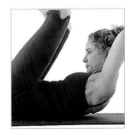

FIG. 2

* Exhale, activating your zipper, hip belt, navel to spine, and triangles to roll your upper body *all* the way up. Empty *all* the air out as you sink the abdominals deeper. Using percussive breathing, inhale twice through your nose and exhale twice through your mouth ("sniff sniff, blow blow"). Perform 10 sets, moving the maximum amount of air through your body with each breath. Work up to 10 sets of breathing in for 5 counts and then out for 5 counts.

OPTIONS

* If you experience tension in your neck, use a hand towel under your upper back and head to provide support, as in Head Float and Rib Slide (see page 89).

BODY SCAN

* Avoid arching your back and pooching your abdominals. This can happen when your legs are too far from your torso.

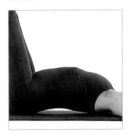

* Avoiding tucking your chin too far in to your chest. Maintain length through your neck.

* Avoid bringing your knees too far in to your body, as this causes your pelvis to tuck.

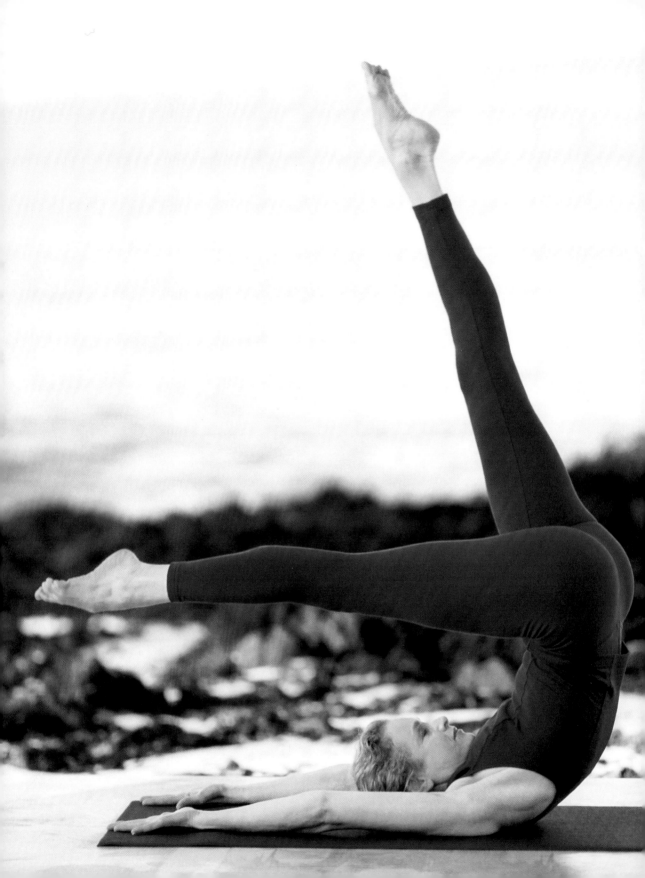

[4]

BEYOND THE BASICS:
CLASSIC MATWORK

Now that you've laid a strong foundation for your Pilates practice with the B.E.A.M. Fundamentals, it's time to introduce you to the exercises based on Joseph Pilates's original matwork routines. Keep in mind, however, that since this is a book for beginners (both beginning exercisers and those unfamiliar with Pilates), the classic mat exercises presented here have been modified from their original—and more difficult—forms.

As I introduce each new classic exercise in this section, where possible I'll remind you which specific B.E.A.M. Fundamental prepared you for the classic exercise you're about to learn. As with the B.E.A.M. Fundamentals, I recommend that you stick as closely as possible to the order presented here and that you don't move on to the next exercise until you've mastered the previous one. The reason for this is that I've designed the workout to stretch and strengthen every part of your body in a particular sequence so as to correct muscular imbalances and improve posture.

This chapter finishes with a roll up to standing posture, so you end this workout in the same way you started in Chapter 2—with a posture check. (I hope your standing posture will have improved!) You'll round out classic matwork with a balance test and will walk away from your workout feeling refreshed and renewed.

BREATHING 100s

If you had gone to Joseph Pilates for a lesson half a century ago, this is the first exercise he would have given you. Breathing 100s work everything: Your abs are engaged, your legs are stretched, your arms are pumping vigorously, and your lungs are fully inflated and deflated with each set. The 100s are invigorating because they send blood coursing through your body. Don't be surprised if you feel hot!

BREATHE

Inhale for 5 counts through your nose, and exhale for 5 counts through your mouth.

ENERGIZE

Accent the first count of each exhalation by drawing navel to spine.

ALIGN

Adjust the angle of your legs in the air in order to maintain scooped abs at all times. (Bend your knees if necessary.)

MOVE

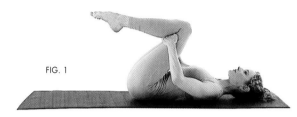

FIG. 1

FIG. 1

✴ Lie on your back with your hands holding the backs of your thighs and your knees bent and squeezed together in parallel stance. Inhale in home position.

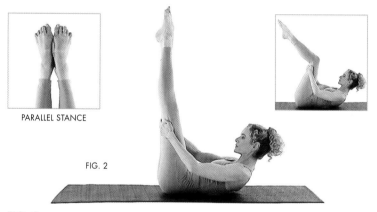

PARALLEL STANCE

FIG. 2

FIG. 2

✴ Exhale completely to extend your legs vertically, simultaneously rolling your upper body into the Rib Slide position from B.E.A.M. Fundamentals (see page 89). Inhale through your nose for 5 rhythmic counts, and exhale through your mouth for 5 counts. Perform 10 sets. If you feel tension in your neck or shoulders, or if your abs are pooching, keep your knees bent.

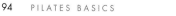

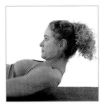
PILATES STANCE

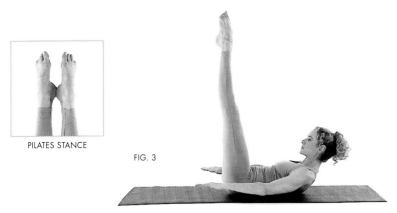
FIG. 3

FIG. 3

✳ If you feel ready for a more challenging position, rotate your thighs open into Pilates stance, and extend your arms horizontally at your sides with your palms facing down. Perform rhythmic arm beats 4 to 6 inches off the mat in time with your breath. The arm beats should be steady, like a metronome, accenting the movement down toward the mat. Initiate the arm beats from the underarm muscles and the back of your shoulders.

 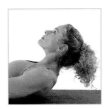

✳ Do not tuck your chin so tightly to your chest that you restrict your breathing (*left*). You should be able to sing while maintaining the position. Don't allow your chin to lift and your head to fall back, as this will strain your neck (*right*).

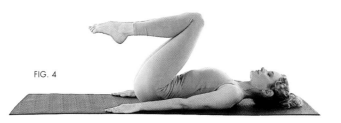
FIG. 4

FIG. 4

✳ After the last set, inhale to roll your upper body down; then exhale to draw your knees in to your chest in home position.

OPTIONS

✳ You can support your head with your hands as in Mini Breathing from B.E.A.M. Fundamentals (see page 90).

✳ For a greater challenge, lower your straight legs toward your mat, maintaining the Rib Slide position without pooching your abs.

BODY SCAN

✳ Draw your shoulders down away from your ears, and avoid hunching.

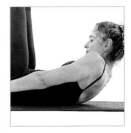

✳ Avoid locking your elbows, as this encourages overuse of your upper shoulder and pectoral muscles.

TRANSITION

✳ Hug your knees and curl your upper body off the mat to roll up to a seated position. Grab your exercise band for Roll Down.

ROLL DOWN

In traditional Pilates matwork, the Roll Up is the next exercise. Since rolling up off the mat against the force of gravity is very challenging, we start here with rolling down onto the mat. If you're unable to control your abdominals throughout the full range of the descent, modify the exercise and roll only partway down until you gain more control.

BREATHE

Inhale in home position, and exhale to roll down. Inhale while lying down, and exhale to roll up.

ENERGIZE

Visualize two-way energy reaching through the crown of your head and out your heels. Visualize your shoulder blades sliding down into your back pockets throughout the exercise.

ALIGN

Sit tall out of your hips with your shoulders drawn down away from your ears.

MOVE

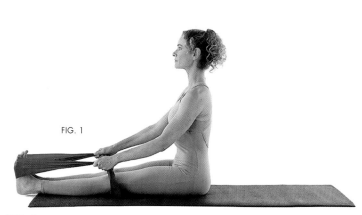

FIG. 1

FIG. 1

✳ Wrap an exercise band around the soles of your flexed feet, holding the ends with extended arms. Hold the band so that it is already taut. (The tension will help you roll back up.) Keep your arms straight without locking your elbows. Squeeze your legs together, and sit tall out of your hips. Inhale in home position.

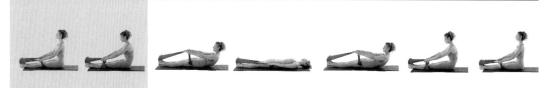

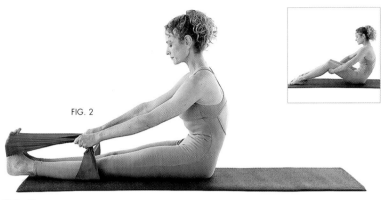

FIG. 2

FIG. 2

❋ Begin exhaling, scooping your abs to form a C shape with your torso. (*Note:* This movement of your pelvis should be identical to Pelvic Tuck and Arch from B.E.A.M. Fundamentals; see page 62.)

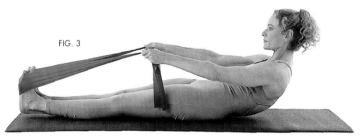

FIG. 3

FIG. 3

❋ Continue to exhale, imprinting your spine one vertebra at a time onto the mat. Be sure to keep your head and neck in line with the rest of your spine. Avoid dropping your head back or tucking your chin tightly toward your chest.

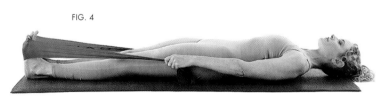

FIG. 4

FIG. 4

❋ Complete the exhalation as you release to neutral spine on the mat, stretching your arms long at your sides. Inhale in neutral. Begin exhaling, tucking your pelvis and rolling your upper torso off the mat (see Fig. 3). Continue peeling your vertebrae off the mat, completing the exhalation as you return to the C shape (see Fig. 2). Inhale to sit tall in home position, and exhale to begin the next Roll Down. Perform 6 repetitions.

OPTIONS

❋ If your abs pooch, modify your starting position by bending your knees and placing your feet hip-width apart on the mat. Hold the backs of your thighs and walk your hands along your thighs as you exhale into the scoop. Roll down only as far as you can maintain scooped abs; then inhale, holding the scoop. Exhale to return to the C shape. Inhale to sit up tall.

BODY SCAN

❋ Be sure to imprint your waistline onto the mat *before* your upper back. Don't lean back through your upper back (shoulders).

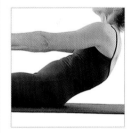

TRANSITION

❋ Perform one last Roll Down, and remain lying on your back. Set your exercise band aside to prepare for Roll Over.

ROLL OVER

Roll Over remains a standard in most Pilates mat classes because it teaches the basic principle of peeling the spine off the mat vertebra by vertebra and then imprinting it back down with ultimate control. You have already practiced this principle in Pelvic Press from B.E.A.M. Fundamentals (see page 68), and the modified version of Roll Over presented here uses precisely the same breathing pattern. You may repeat Pelvic Press in place of Roll Over if you have tight lower back muscles or if you experience any upper back or neck discomfort when rolling.

BREATHE

Exhale when articulating the spine.

ENERGIZE

Form a strong tripod with the back of your arms stretched long at your sides and the back of your head and shoulders pressed firmly into the mat.

ALIGN

In the open leg position, feet should be slightly wider than hip-width apart.

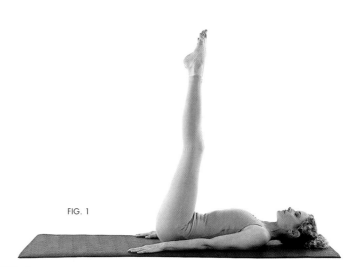

FIG. 1

FIG. 1

✻ Press your legs firmly together, keeping them parallel and aligned vertically over your hips. Keep your knees slightly bent, and point your feet. Inhale in home position.

MOVE

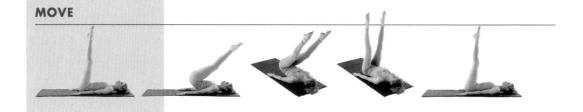

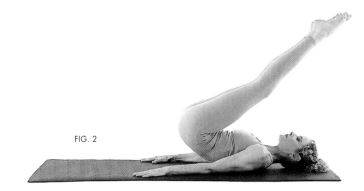

FIG. 2

FIG. 2

✳ Exhale to tuck your pelvis, peeling your spine off the mat vertebra by vertebra, beginning with your tailbone. Be sure to initiate the Roll Over by tucking your pelvis from your lowest abdominals. Angle your legs diagonally above your head.

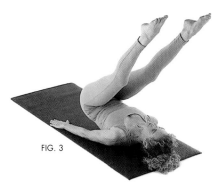

FIG. 3

FIG. 3

✳ Inhale, holding the top of the Roll Over and opening your legs just beyond hip-width apart.

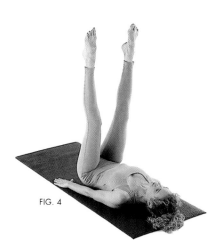

FIG. 4

FIG. 4

✳ Exhale, imprinting your spine back down on the mat one vertebra at a time. As your legs become vertical, inhale to close them, returning to home position. Perform 4 Roll Overs, and then reverse the leg pattern for 4 more, this time peeling your spine off with open legs and imprinting down with closed legs.

OPTIONS

✳ For a greater challenge, straighten your legs fully and roll up higher onto your upper back, angling your legs parallel to the floor.

BODY SCAN

✳ Avoid collapsing your thighs onto your chest as you imprint your spine back toward the mat.

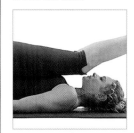

✳ Do *not* initiate Roll Over by swinging your legs overhead.

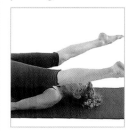

TRANSITION

✳ After your final Roll Over, hug your knees in to your chest for a good stretch.

LEG CIRCLES

Knee Stirs, from B.E.A.M. Fundamentals (see page 60), prepared you for Leg Circles. Both exercises use identical breathing patterns. Stabilize your pelvis by engaging your Powerhouse, and keep your circles small, precise, and rhythmic.

BREATHE

Inhale with long and sustained breaths as your leg begins to circle; exhale with short and percussive breaths to accent the return to home position.

ENERGIZE

Visualize two-way energy coming out of the crown of your head and the heel of your supporting leg.

ALIGN

Align your leg on the mat directly under your hip. Keep the imaginary belt stretched across your abdomen from hip to hip level at all times.

MOVE

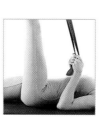

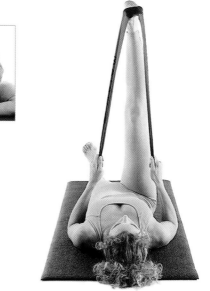

FIG. 1

FIG. 1

* Place a pillow under your head or neck, and wrap an exercise band around your right foot. Raise your right leg into the air, aligning it vertically over your hip. Press your elbows firmly into the mat to stabilize your torso. It's tempting to tuck the pelvis here, but be sure to maintain a neutral spine. Modify the position as needed if tight hips and hamstrings limit your range of motion. Exhale in home position.

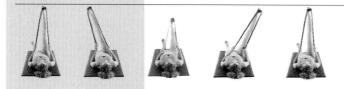

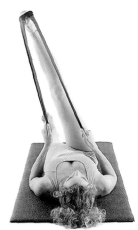

FIG. 2

FIG. 2

* Begin inhaling as you bring your right leg across your body toward your left shoulder.

* To facilitate maintaining a neutral spine, bend both knees as needed and extend your arms long at your sides.

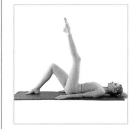

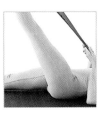

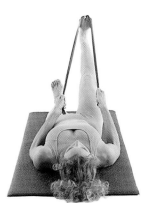

FIG. 3

FIG. 3

* Complete the inhalation as you sweep your leg down and away from you. Begin exhaling as your leg crosses the midline of your body.

BODY SCAN

* To avoid rocking your torso from side to side, engage your abs and the smile muscle of the supporting leg to enhance your stability.

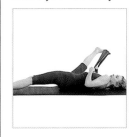

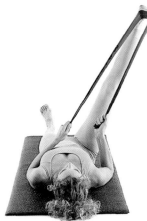

FIG. 4

FIG. 4

* Continue exhaling as your leg circles open to the right. Keep your left hip anchored firmly to the mat. Complete the exhalation as you accent the return to home position. Perform 6 circles; then change direction for 6 more, opening your leg out to the right and then circling down and across your body to return to home position. Keep the circles small at first, concentrating on anchoring your pelvis in neutral position. Switch legs, and perform 6 circles in each direction.

TRANSITION

* Release the exercise band, and bring both knees in to your chest. Hold the backs of your thighs. Roll your upper body up, and come to a seated position at the front edge of your mat for Rolling Like a Ball.

ROLLING LIKE A BALL

Joseph Pilates believed rolling to be extremely beneficial to the body for several reasons. First, it promotes an even, balanced flexibility of the spinal column. Second, the cerebro-spinal fluid, which bathes and protects the spine and the intervertebral discs, circulates more freely with this kind of active "massage" to the spine. Third and finally, Pilates believed that his deep breathing, combined with the rolling and unrolling of the spine, cleanses the lungs of impurities and stimulates a sluggish digestive tract.

BREATHE

Quickly inhale in home position; exhale in two parts to roll back and recover. Be sure to exhale completely as you roll, and inhale dynamically as you balance for a moment in home position.

ENERGIZE

Experiment with just the right amount of attack and energy to roll, and recover to hover for a moment as you inhale quickly, only to roll again.

ALIGN

Paint an imaginary highway line down the center of your mat, and roll your spine exactly like a wheel over the line. There should be no bumps or swerving on your road!

MOVE

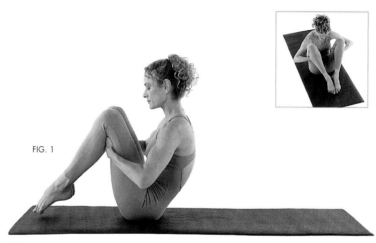

FIG. 1

FIG. 1

✳ Place yourself at the front edge of your mat. Hover in a rounded C shape, sitting just behind the sitting bones. Grasp the backs of your thighs, hovering your toes just off the mat. Inhale percussively through your nose.

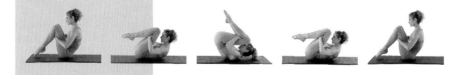

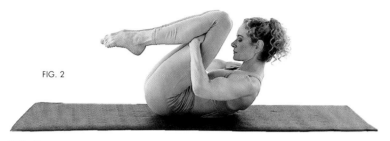

FIG. 2

FIG. 2

* Keep your chin tucked toward your chest and begin exhaling as you roll backward. Maintain the same distance between your heels and your buttocks throughout the roll, holding a tight ball shape.

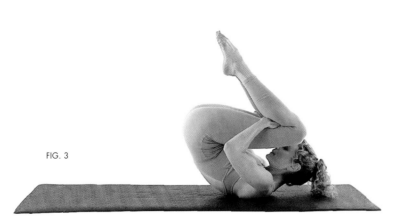

FIG. 3

FIG. 3

* Continue exhaling as you roll back onto your shoulders. Roll onto the backs of your shoulders at the farthest point of your roll. Avoid rolling up onto your neck. Then reverse your roll, returning to home position as you continue to empty your lungs completely. Hover in home position for a moment as you inhale percussively to repeat the roll. Work up to 10 repetitions.

OPTIONS

* As you advance, grasp your ankles, creating a tighter ball shape.

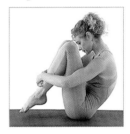

BODY SCAN

* Avoid pumping your heels back and forward to gain momentum.

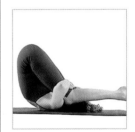

TRANSITION

* After completing the last roll, rest your feet down. Move your hands behind you to the center of your mat. Scoot your buttocks back between your hands.

* Grasp the backs of your thighs and scoop your abs as you exhale. Roll slowly down onto your back for Single Leg Stretch.

SINGLE LEG STRETCH

Pistons, from the B.E.A.M. Fundamentals (see page 66), are the preparation for this classic mat exercise. You can perform Single Leg Stretch with many different breathing patterns and at varying speeds. It will test your coordination, as well as the flexibility of your hips, knees, and lower back. And, of course, there is the abdominal work built into any Pilates exercise!

BREATHE

Inhale as your knees pass one another; exhale to fold the opposite knee in to your chest.

ENERGIZE

Imagine you are holding a filled-to-the-brim teacup balanced on your lower belly as you perform this exercise. Don't spill a drop!

ALIGN

Pay attention to your hands: If your right knee is bent, place your right hand on your right ankle and your left hand on your right knee. As you change legs, reverse your hand position.

MOVE

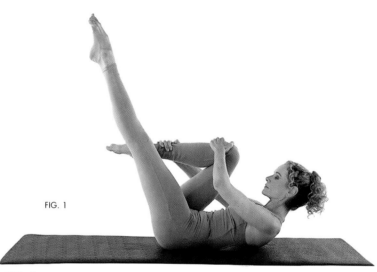

FIG. 1

FIG. 1

✳ Exhale to roll your head and shoulders up off the mat. Fold your right knee in to your chest, right hand to right ankle, left hand to right knee. Extend your left leg into the air at an angle you can hold without pooching your abs.

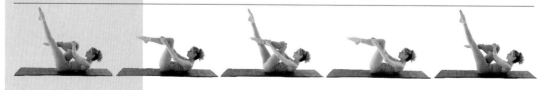

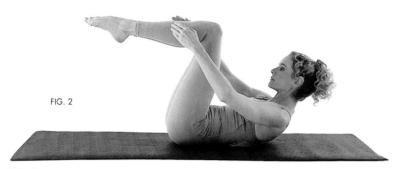

FIG. 2

FIG. 2

❋ Inhale as you draw your left leg back toward your chest and your knees pass one another, maintaining the curl in your upper body.

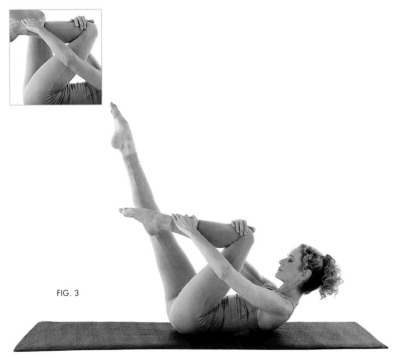

FIG. 3

FIG. 3

❋ Exhale to fold your left knee in to your chest, left hand to left ankle, right hand to left knee, extending your right leg into the air. Perform 5 repetitions with each leg, alternating legs.

OPTIONS

❋ If your neck strains easily, support your head with your hands.

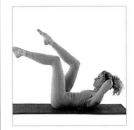

❋ When you feel ready, repeat a second set with flexed feet, pushing out through your heels using your smile muscles.

BODY SCAN

❋ Stay within the frame of your body and keep your legs parallel.

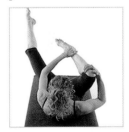

TRANSITION

❋ Fold both knees in to your chest and rest your head down for a moment. Then exhale as you roll up to a seated position at the front edge of your mat for Spine Stretch.

SPINE STRETCH

Spine Stretch is a personal favorite of mine. I love that it begins upright, tests the flexibility of the spine in a forward bend, and then gives you the opportunity to restack the vertebrae one on top of the other back in the upright posture. When you're learning Spine Stretch for the first time, practice it slowly. Once you feel you're performing it correctly, start speeding up without losing your form. This way, you'll train your muscles to spring back to ideal posture from "muscle memory," a well-known technique of professional dancers and athletes.

BREATHE

Inhale in home position and in your maximum forward bend position. Exhale as you're rolling down or up the spine.

ENERGIZE

Imagine you're seated against a wall for this exercise. Your spine is wallpaper that alternately peels away from and is pasted back up on the wall. No wrinkles should appear in your wallpaper!

ALIGN

Sit up tall out of your hips, and align your shoulders vertically over your hips.

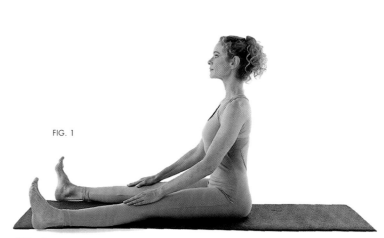

FIG. 1

FIG. 1

✳ Open your legs in a small V, with bent or straight legs as needed. Flex your feet, reach out of your heels, and pull your imaginary marionette string to sit tall out of your hips. Drop your shoulder blades into your back pockets, lengthen your neck, and level your eyes straight ahead. Inhale in home position.

MOVE

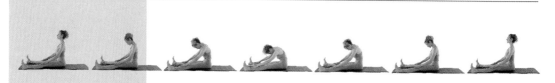

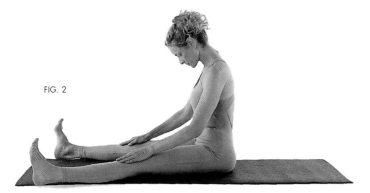

FIG. 2

FIG. 2

* Begin exhaling, dropping your chin toward your chest.

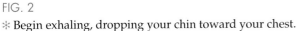

FIG. 3

FIG. 3

* Continue exhaling, letting a heavy head take you into a slow roll down, vertebra by vertebra. Slide the palms of your hands along the tops of your legs as you descend.

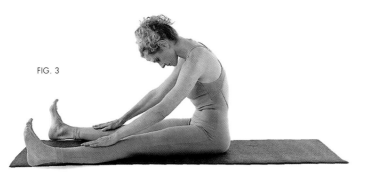

FIG. 4

FIG. 4

* Complete the exhalation as you arrive at full stretch. Maintain the scoop in your abs, and be sure your buttocks remain anchored to the floor. Inhale, holding the scoop. Exhale to restack the vertebrae, one on top of the other, back to home position. Perform 6 to 8 repetitions.

OPTIONS

* If your hamstrings and lower back are tight, sit on a pillow and bend your knees.

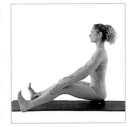

* Try this exercise seated with your back against a wall.

BODY SCAN

* Begin the Spine Stretch by dropping your head first.

* Avoid hinging forward from your hips; that gives you a great hamstring stretch, but it doesn't stretch your spine!

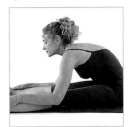

TRANSITION

* After the last stretch, bring your feet together at the front of the mat for Spine Twist.

SPINE TWIST

Rotating the spine is an action we all do every day, but usually we aren't thinking about maintaining proper form while we do it. Back injuries often occur while twisting, so it's extremely important to learn how to do it correctly. Whenever you begin a twist, remember to lengthen your spine vertically first so that you unload the downward pressure on your intervertebral discs and spinal cord. Then, as you rotate, keep the movement smooth and controlled, with equal effort placed on sitting tall as you spiral around.

BREATHE

Inhale to rotate, and exhale to return to center.

ENERGIZE

Visualize three energy lines traveling through your body: one out the crown of your head to the ceiling, the second out your heels, and the third from elbow to elbow across your chest.

ALIGN

Keep your shoulders and ribs in an even horizontal line at all times. (It's tempting to collapse on one side as you rotate your torso.)

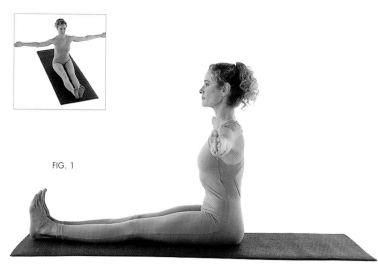

FIG. 1

FIG. 1

✳ Keep your legs straight and feet flexed, or bend your knees as needed to sit up tall out of your hips. Bring both arms up to your sides at shoulder height, palms facing forward. Exhale all of your air in home position.

MOVE

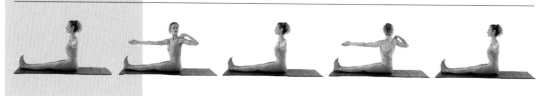

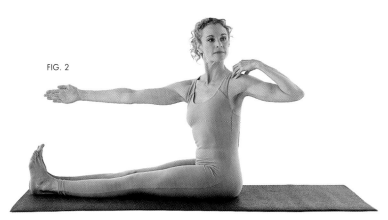

FIG. 2

FIG. 2

✳ Place the fingertips of your left hand on your left shoulder as you inhale percussively twice through your nose to rotate left. Avoid jerky or abrupt twisting motions. Energy stretches across your chest from shoulder to shoulder. Drop your shoulder blades down into your back pockets, and keep your headlights facing front. Exhale to return to home position.

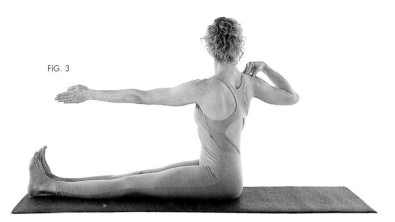

FIG. 3

FIG. 3

✳ Inhale to change hands and rotate to the right. Exhale to return to home position. Perform 5 repetitions.

OPTIONS

✳ For a simpler version, place the fingertips of both hands on your shoulders. Keep your elbows open to shoulder height.

✳ If your hamstrings and lower back are tight, sit on a pillow and bend your knees.

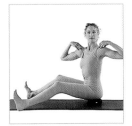

BODY SCAN

✳ Feel an imaginary marionette string pulling the energy up from the base of your spine through the top of your head.

✳ Rotate around your center *without* falling off your vertical line.

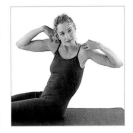

TRANSITION

✳ Turn facedown on the mat for Back Leg and Arm Extensions.

BACK LEG AND ARM EXTENSIONS

Back Leg and Arm Extensions combine to form the classic mat exercise Swimming. Although we've practiced Back Extensions in the B.E.A.M. Fundamentals (see page 78), here we add arm and leg movements to this all-important back strengthener. As always, begin slowly, paying particular attention to proper form, and then speed up as your skills improve.

BREATHE

Inhale to prepare by lengthening your body in home position. Exhale to lift.

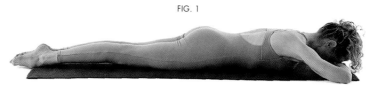

FIG. 1

FIG. 1

❋ Lie facedown on the mat, feet hip-width apart. Stack your hands under your forehead. Inhale to extend your body long, and engage your Powerhouse to stabilize the torso in home position. Visualize your shoulder blades moving down into your back pockets.

ENERGIZE

Feel marionette strings pulling the tips of your toes to the wall behind you. The image here is to lengthen your legs out of your hips without overarching your lower back.

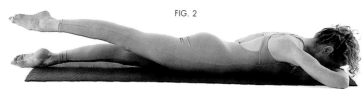

FIG. 2

FIG. 2

❋ Exhale to lengthen your right leg off the mat. Keep a long line from the base of your buttocks out through your toes. Inhale to return to home.

ALIGN

Your legs should be hip-width apart to begin. (Later, you may narrow your legs closer together.) Your arms should be at least shoulder-width apart to reduce upper shoulder tension.

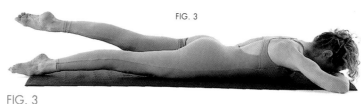

FIG. 3

FIG. 3

❋ Exhale to lift your left leg; inhale to return home. Perform 4 or 5 sets.

MOVE

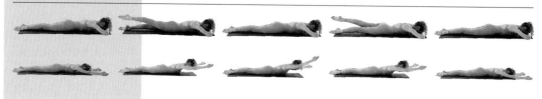

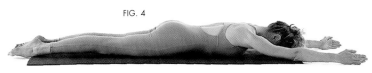

FIG. 4

* Lying facedown, extend your arms out to form a V. Keep your feet hip-width apart. Exhale completely.

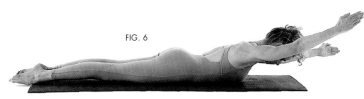

FIG. 5

* Inhale to engage your Powerhouse and draw your shoulder blades down into your back pockets as you raise your entire upper body slightly off the floor, hovering in an extended position. Your shoulders should remain level as your arms extend.

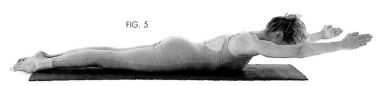

FIG. 6

* Exhale to lift your right arm; inhale to return to the hover with both arms even (see Fig. 5).

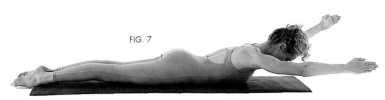

FIG. 7

* Exhale to lift your left arm; inhale to return to the hover. Perform 4 or 5 sets, and then exhale to relax to home position.

OPTIONS

* If your neck strains easily or you feel pressure in your lower back, place a cushion under your hips, keep your forehead resting on a pillow, and perform only the arm movements.

BODY SCAN

* Avoid lifting your leg too high and over-arching your lower back.

* Keep your head-lights and pubic bone pressed firmly into the mat.

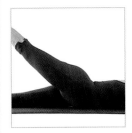

* Keep the back of your neck long, and focus your eyes on your mat.

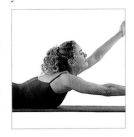

TRANSITION

* Remain lying face-down for Swimming.

SWIMMING

We will now combine Back Leg and Arm Extensions into Swimming. Most students find this exercise challenging for two reasons. First, it requires coordinating the contralateral movement of arms and legs moving in opposition, as in walking. Second, it requires strong core muscles to work the arms and legs simultaneously against the force of gravity. Begin slowly, paying attention to proper form, and speed up as your skill improves.

BREATHE

Inhale to prepare by lengthening your body in home position. Exhale to lift.

FIG. 1

FIG. 1

* Lying facedown, extend your arms out to form a V. Your feet should remain hip-width apart. Exhale completely.

ENERGIZE

Feel marionette strings pulling the tips of your fingers and toes to the walls in front of you and behind you. The idea here is to lengthen the body, not to lift your arms and legs!

ALIGN

Position your arms at least shoulder-width apart to reduce upper shoulder tension. Your legs should be hip-width apart to begin. (Later, you may narrow your legs closer together.)

MOVE

FIG. 2

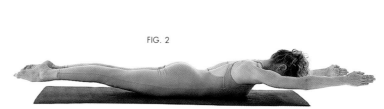

FIG. 2

* Inhale to engage your Powerhouse and draw your shoulder blades down into your back pockets as you raise both your upper body and legs slightly off the floor, hovering in an extended position.

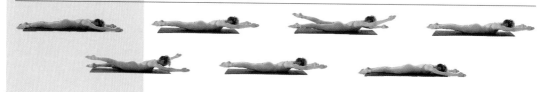

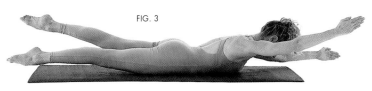

FIG. 3

FIG. 3

❊ Exhale to lift your right arm and left leg. Inhale to return to the hover with your arms and legs level.

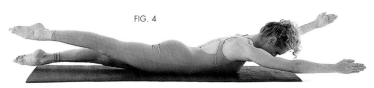

FIG. 4

FIG. 4

❊ Exhale to lift your left arm and right leg. Inhale to return to the hover. Perform 4 or 5 sets, and then exhale to lengthen your entire body as you release to home position.

OPTIONS

❊ If your neck strains easily or you feel pressure in your lower back, keep your forehead resting on a pillow and perform only the arm movements.

❊ Use a pillow under your hips if you feel pressure in your lower back.

❊ When you feel ready, speed up your Swimming and flutter kick using quick, percussive breathing, in for 2 counts and out for 2 counts.

BODY SCAN

❊ Avoid rolling from side to side as you switch arms and legs.

❊ Keep the back of your neck long and your Powerhouse strong.

TRANSITION

❊ Press your buttocks to your heels in Rest Position (see page 82). Relax your forehead into the mat, and release your neck muscles. If your neck feels strained, stack your fists under your forehead.

FRONT LEG EXTENSIONS AND MODIFIED TEASER

Front Leg Extensions prepare you for the classic mat exercise called Teaser. In a traditional mat class, these exercises are considered advanced, but I've presented them here in easier, modified versions that will strengthen your abdominals and help trim your waistline.

BREATHE

Inhale to extend your legs; exhale to bend your knees. Exhale to tuck your pelvis, drawing your legs slightly closer to your torso. Inhale to release to the Leg Extension position.

ENERGIZE

Feel as though contracting your abs into the backs of your hands as you exhale is the impetus to bend your knees. Perform Pelvic Tuck and Arch (see page 62) to initiate the Teaser.

ALIGN

Everyone's proportions are different. If you have a short torso and long legs, the angle at which you extend your legs will be more vertical than if you have shorter legs and a long torso.

MOVE

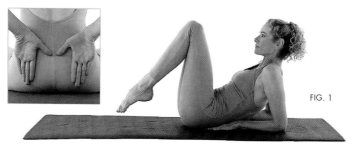

FIG. 1

FIG. 1

✳ Come to a semireclined position with your hands tucked under your pelvis, palms facing down. Bend your knees and press them tightly together, toes hovering above the mat. Exhale completely in home position.

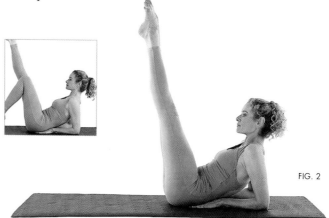

FIG. 2

FIG. 2

✳ Inhale to extend both legs simultaneously, without moving your thighs. Exhale to tuck your pelvis and return to home position. Initiate the knee bend with a deep contraction of your abdominals. Another option is to alternate extending first one leg, then the other, without moving your thighs. Perform 5 to 10 repetitions.

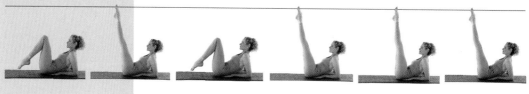

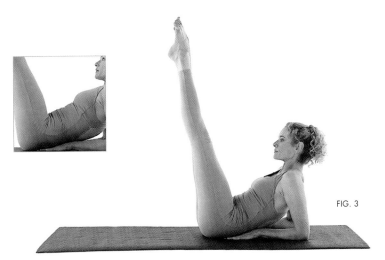

FIG. 3

FIG. 3

✳ To perform Modified Teaser, begin from the last Leg Extension you performed, in a semireclined position with your hands tucked under your pelvis, palms facing down. Extend your legs and press your thighs tightly together in home position.

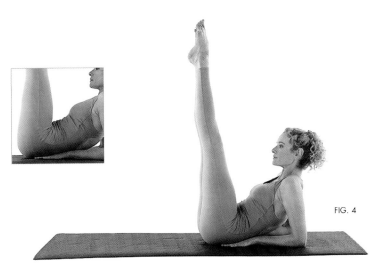

FIG. 4

FIG. 4

✳ Exhale to tuck your pelvis, pressing into your hands. Your legs will move slightly closer to you, but avoid pulling your thighs in from your hip sockets! Inhale to release. Keep the movement of your legs minimal. The pelvic tuck dictates the leg movement. Experiment with slightly different placements of the palms of your hands under your pelvis, and find the optimum position for you. You should definitely feel a slight downward pressure onto the backs of your hands when you tuck your pelvis, but it should *not* be painful. Perform 5 to 10 repetitions.

OPTIONS

✳ If your lower back strains easily, bend your knees as needed.

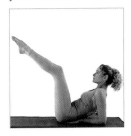

BODY SCAN

✳ If you extend your legs too low, your belly will pooch.

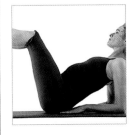

✳ Avoid collapsing your upper body. Push up out of your forearms.

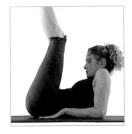

TRANSITION

✳ Grab your exercise band and roll onto your back for Pendulum.

PENDULUM

Pendulum evolves directly from the B.E.A.M. Fundamentals exercise Cross-Leg Fall (see page 70). Like Cross-Leg Fall, it's wonderful for the oblique abdominals but avoids strain in your upper neck and shoulders. Pendulum is also a direct preparation for the classic mat exercise Corkscrew.

BREATHE

Inhale to shift your pelvis to one side. Exhale to return to center.

ENERGIZE

Visualize your upper body glued to the mat as your lower body shifts from side to side.

ALIGN

Your legs should be raised to 90 degrees or more throughout the exercise, to reduce stress on your lower back.

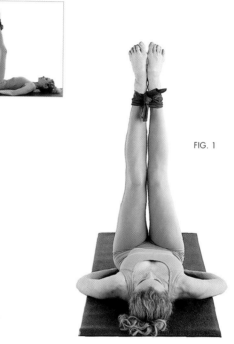

FIG. 1

FIG. 1

✳ Place a small pillow under your head or neck. Tie an exercise band around your ankles, and extend your legs toward the ceiling, keeping your knees relaxed. Place your hands under your pelvis, palms down. Exhale completely in home position.

MOVE

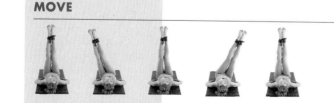

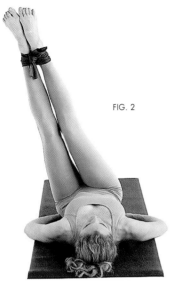

FIG. 2

✳ Inhale to shift your weight into your left buttock and pelvis. Keep your inner thighs pressed together firmly, as if you had only one leg. Exhale, imprinting your spine from the top down, into home position.

FIG. 2

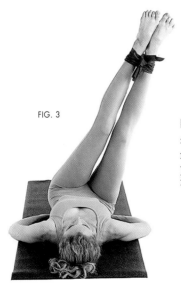

FIG. 3

FIG. 3

✳ Inhale to shift your weight into your right buttock and pelvis. Exhale, imprinting your spine from the top down, into home position. Perform 4 or 5 sets.

OPTIONS

✳ Place a pillow under your hips, and loop an exercise band around the soles of both feet. Stretch your legs vertically, keeping your knees relaxed.

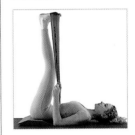

BODY SCAN

✳ Visualize a highway line running straight down the middle of your mat, and imprint your spine back onto it, diagonally from top to bottom, each time you return to home position.

✳ Maintain your upper body and neck in neutral alignment.

✳ Avoid engaging your hips and buttocks to move the pelvis. Focus on the diagonal action of your obliques to level your pelvis.

TRANSITION

✳ Remain in home position to begin Corkscrew.

CORKSCREW

This classic exercise is considered superadvanced by Pilates purists, but it is presented here in a simpler, modified form. The breathing pattern remains faithful to the original, however, so when you feel ready to advance your Pilates workout, you'll already be familiar with this fabulous exercise.

BREATHE

Inhale as you shift your weight to one side. Hold your breath as you circle your legs away from you. Exhale as your legs cross the midline of your body and complete the corkscrew.

ENERGIZE

Control your exhale from the center of your abdomen, as if you're slowly letting the air out of a balloon. When you arrive back home, empty the rest of your air out in one strong blast.

ALIGN

Keep your circles small, precise, and equal from side to side. Return to a centered home position each time.

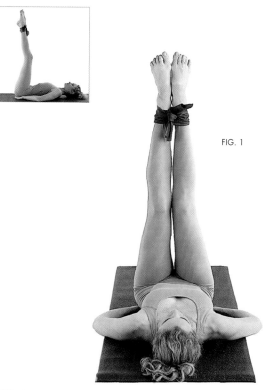

FIG. 1

FIG. 1

✳ Lie on your back with an exercise band around your ankles, your legs vertical, and your knees slightly bent. Place a small pillow under your head or neck. Exhale in home position.

MOVE

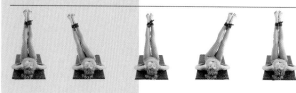

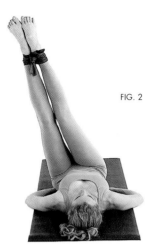

FIG. 2

FIG. 2

✳ Inhale as you shift your weight onto your left buttock and pelvis, allowing your legs to follow along to the left.

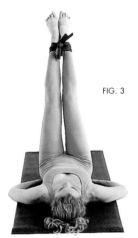

FIG. 3

FIG. 3

✳ Hold your inhale as you sweep your legs down and away from you, circling them back through the midline of your body.

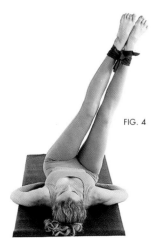

FIG. 4

FIG. 4

✳ As your legs cross the midline of your body, exhale percussively to shift your weight onto your right buttock and pelvis. Allow your legs to follow along to the right and complete your circle with a strong contraction of your abs to finish in home position (see Fig. 1). Repeat Corkscrew in the opposite direction. Work up to 5 sets.

OPTIONS

✳ Place a pillow under your hips, and loop an exercise band around the soles of both feet. Stretch your legs vertically, keeping your knees relaxed.

BODY SCAN

✳ As your legs circle down and away, take care not to overarch your spine and pooch your abs.

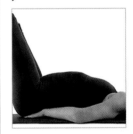

TRANSITION

✳ Turn onto your left side for Side Leg Kicks.

SIDE LEG KICKS

Now that you understand the principle of maintaining a neutral spine while lying on your back or stomach, the next six exercises will challenge your stability in the side lying position. This series is great for toning your inner and outer thighs, hips, and buttocks. Perform all of the next six exercises on one side; then switch sides and repeat the entire series.

BREATHE

Double inhale ("sniff sniff") through your nose as your leg sweeps forward, and give one long exhalation through your mouth as your leg sweeps back.

ENERGIZE

Visualize that your torso is in a body cast from your shoulders to the top of your hip joints, so only the working leg can move in this exercise.

ALIGN

Check often to see if your top hip is aligned evenly over the bottom one.

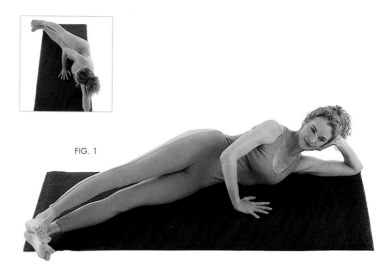

FIG. 1

FIG. 1

✳ Align your left elbow, shoulder, and hip with the back edge of your mat. Extend both legs to the front edge of your mat, and flex your feet. Prop your left arm under your head. Place your right hand on the floor in front of your rib cage in home position.

MOVE

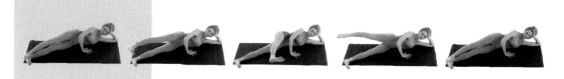

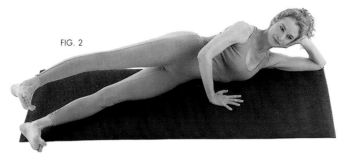

FIG. 2

FIG. 2

✳ Exhale all the air out of your lungs before you begin, and lift your right leg to hip height.

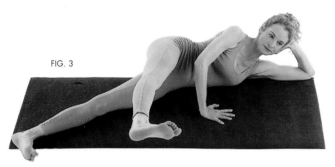

FIG. 3

FIG. 3

✳ Inhale to kick front, pulsing forward twice and using percussive "sniff sniff" breathing.

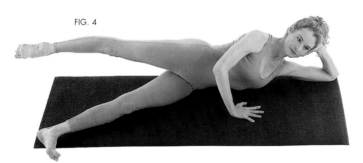

FIG. 4

FIG. 4

✳ Blow all the air out in a long exhalation as you sweep your leg back with a pointed foot. Trace a steady arc, reaching long out of your hip. Work up to 10 repetitions.

OPTIONS

✳ Bend your bottom leg in front. Relax your head on a pillow with your bottom arm extended.

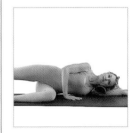

BODY SCAN

✳ Kicking your leg too far forward will round your back.

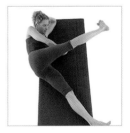

✳ Kicking your leg too far back will over-arch your back.

TRANSITION

✳ Stay on your left side in home position for Side Lying Leg Lifts and Power Circles.

SIDE LYING LEG LIFTS AND POWER CIRCLES

Side Lying Leg Lifts continue our side lying series, focusing on toning and strengthening the muscles of the outer thigh. Done correctly and purposefully, they will help to form a "cut" at the top of your outer thigh where it meets your buttocks. Power Circles are quick, tiny, and precise circles that follow directly after Side Lying Leg Lifts. The work comes entirely from your hip, while your torso remains stable.

BREATHE

For Leg Lifts, exhale to lift your leg, and inhale to lower it.

For Power Circles, inhale for 2 circles and exhale for 2 circles, using the "sniff sniff" breathing pattern.

ENERGIZE

Feel as though you're trying to touch an object just beyond the reach of your foot as you raise and lower your leg with control.

ALIGN

Use your Powerhouse and the arm placed in front of you on the mat to help stabilize your torso as your leg circles. Keep your elbow out and shoulder down on your supporting arm.

MOVE

FIG. 1

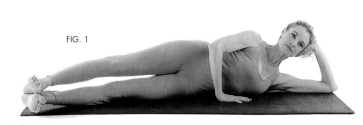

FIG. 1

☀ Align your left elbow, shoulder, and hip with the back edge of your mat. Extend both legs to the front edge of your mat, and flex your feet. Prop your left arm under your head. Place your right hand on the floor in front of your rib cage. Inhale in home position.

FIG. 2

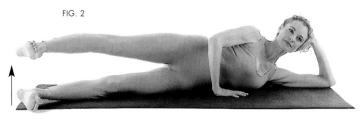

FIG. 2

☀ Exhale to lift your flexed foot to hip height. Keep your leg lifts small and precise, emphasizing length rather than height.

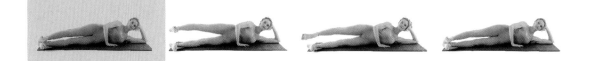

FIG. 3

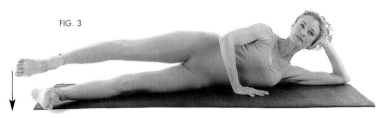

FIG. 3

✳ Point your foot in the lifted position, lengthening out of your hip, and inhale as you slowly lower your leg. Flex your foot again, and exhale to lift. Perform 8 repetitions. Hold the last Leg Lift in the air with a pointed foot for Power Circles.

FIG. 4

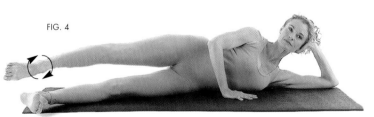

FIG. 4

✳ Begin circling the leg as you inhale. Perform 16 circles in each direction. Imagine a power drill on the end of your foot—lengthen out of the hip to "drill" with your toes. Inhale for 2 circles and exhale for 2 circles, using the "sniff sniff, blow blow" breathing pattern.

OPTIONS

✳ Bend your bottom leg in front of you, and relax your head onto a pillow with your bottom arm extended.

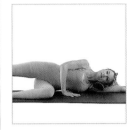

BODY SCAN

✳ Lifting your leg too high will displace the alignment of your pelvis and torso.

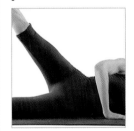

✳ Stabilize your upper body so that it doesn't sway with your leg movements. Your upper body remains quiet as your leg moves from your hip socket.

TRANSITION

✳ Return to home position, and remain on your side for Inner Thigh Leg Lifts and Power Circles.

INNER THIGH LEG LIFTS AND POWER CIRCLES

These exercises focus on strengthening and toning the muscles at the top of your inner thighs.

FIG. 1

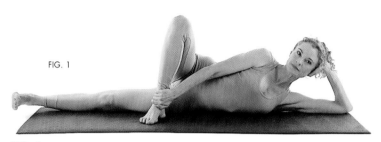

FIG. 1

* Bend your right leg over your left, and grasp your right ankle with your right hand. Move your left leg directly underneath your hip, and flex your foot. Inhale in home position.

FIG. 2

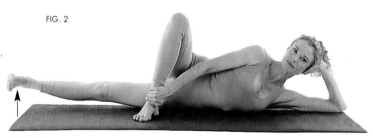

FIG. 2

* Exhale to lengthen and lift your bottom leg. Engage your pelvic floor muscles each time you lift your leg.

BREATHE

For Leg Lifts, exhale to lift, and inhale to lower your leg.

For Power Circles, inhale for 2 circles and exhale for 2 circles, using the "sniff sniff" breathing pattern.

ENERGIZE

Imagine you're keeping an object balanced on the inside of your anklebone as you raise and lower your leg.

ALIGN

Keep your working leg parallel to the floor and directly under your hip.

MOVE

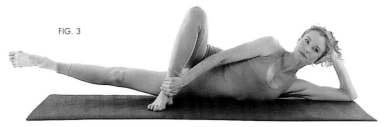

FIG. 3

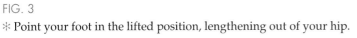

FIG. 3

✳ Point your foot in the lifted position, lengthening out of your hip.

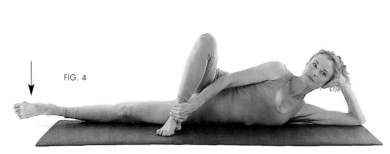

FIG. 4

FIG. 4

✳ Inhale as you slowly lower your leg. Flex your foot again, and exhale to lift. Perform 8 repetitions. Hold the last Leg Lift in the air for Power Circles.

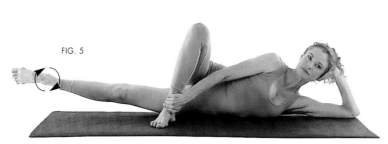

FIG. 5

FIG. 5

✳ Perform 8 Power Circles in each direction, using the "sniff sniff, blow blow" breathing pattern. After your last circle, return to home position.

OPTIONS

✳ Bend your top leg in front, supported by a pillow under your knee.

✳ Relax your head on a pillow with your bottom arm extended.

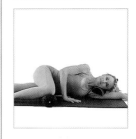

✳ Angle your working leg slightly in front of you at first. As you get stronger, bring your leg more in line with your hip.

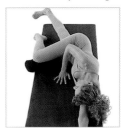

BODY SCAN

✳ Imagine a line of energy extending from the crown of your head down through your body and out the heel of your working leg.

TRANSITION

✳ Stay on your side for Side Lying Quad Stretch.

SIDE LYING QUAD STRETCH

Sitting for long periods of time shortens your hip flexors—the muscles that run along the front of your hips from torso to thigh. Repetitive actions such as running and climbing (and even step aerobics) can also tighten the quads and hip flexors. Much of our Pilates matwork up until now has emphasized flexing the knees in toward the chest, which is great work for the abs and stretches the spine beautifully, but it contributes to tight hip flexors. Now it's time to counter all of this with a good stretch for your hip and quadriceps muscles.

BREATHE

Inhale to back off the stretch just slightly; exhale to deepen it.

ENERGIZE

Imagine that your thigh muscles attach from your navel all the way down to your knee. Do your best to keep your navel and knee in one long, straight line.

ALIGN

Lift your abs to prevent your lower back from overarching and maintain neutral spine.

FIG. 1

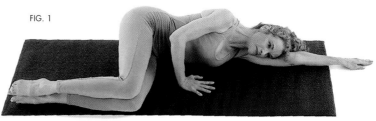

FIG. 1

❋ On your left side, bend both legs in front of you.

MOVE

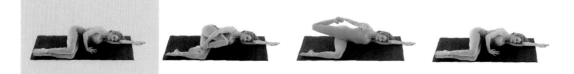

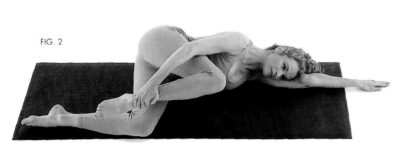

FIG. 2

* Draw your right knee in to your chest and grasp your right ankle with your right hand. Inhale.

OPTIONS

* If you can't reach your back foot with your hand, loop an exercise band around your foot and hold the ends of the band in your hand.

BODY SCAN

* Keep your bottom leg bent at 90 degrees to your torso.

* Keep your top hip, knee, and foot on a level plane.

* Avoid overarching your lower back and pooching your abs.

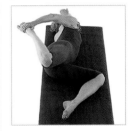

TRANSITION

* Now, return to page 120 and turn onto your right side to complete the Side Lying series on the other side. When completed, come to a seated position for Mermaid.

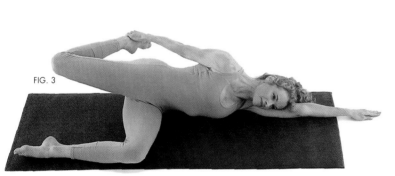

FIG. 3

* As you exhale, draw your thigh down and away from you. Engage your abs and tilt your pubic bone forward and up. Don't overarch your lower back, and remember to breathe! Hold the Quad Stretch for at least 3 to 5 long breath cycles.

MERMAID

This is an elegant exercise that will help you to lengthen and strengthen your lateral obliques, the muscles that help to form your waistline. In everyday life, the lateral obliques are seldom worked, giving rise to the infamous "love handles" and "spare tire" around the midsection. So stretch away, and enjoy the yawning sensation of waking up these under-used muscles!

BREATHE

Inhale to stretch up and over in one direction. Exhale to move into the counter stretch to the other side.

ENERGIZE

Visualize a marionette string pulling you toward the ceiling in home position. Then picture the string pulling you in an upward, arcing motion to create the curve of the side stretch.

ALIGN

Keep your shoulders and hips horizontal, and make sure they stay in home position. Be sure your ribs are not poking out to one side because you're seated on one hip.

MOVE

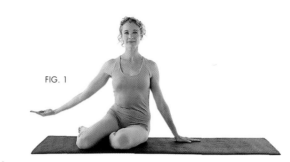

FIG. 1

FIG. 1

* Sit on your left hip with your legs folded to the right side. Place the palm of your left hand on the floor beside your left hip and let your right arm form a gentle arc out to the side, palm up. Exhale and lengthen up out of your hips and through the crown of your head.

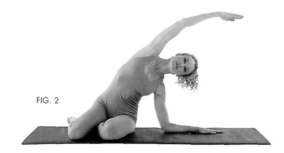

FIG. 2

FIG. 2

* Inhale as you raise your right arm overhead alongside your right ear, stretching as far as you can over to your left side. Your left elbow bends, but don't worry if it doesn't reach the mat. Be sure to lift up through your torso to allow more space for side bending.

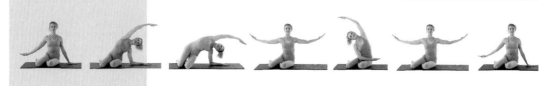

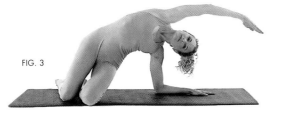

FIG. 3

FIG. 3

Note: This next step, the side lift, is optional. If you don't feel ready, then move on to Fig. 4.

✳ Continue inhaling as you raise your left hip off the mat by driving your left forearm into the floor. Create one long, graceful arc from your right hip to your fingertips.

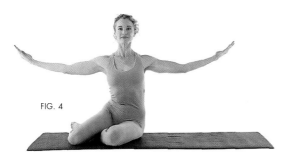

FIG. 4

FIG. 4

✳ Holding your inhalation, come back to the vertical position with your arms at shoulder height, palms up. Pass through this position, keeping the movement flowing. Each time you pass through vertical alignment, be sure your shoulders are aligned squarely over your hips for an instant.

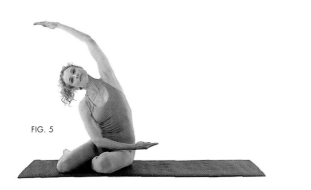

FIG. 5

FIG. 5

✳ Exhale to reverse the curve, raising your left arm overhead. Bring your right arm in front of your waist as you stretch to the right. Perform 3 to 5 Mermaids on each side.

OPTIONS

✳ If you have tight hips or feel pressure in your knee, place a pillow under the hip you're seated on.

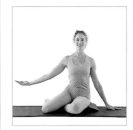

✳ The optional side lift will strengthen your upper body and shoulders, preparing you for more rigorous exercises.

BODY SCAN

✳ Imagine your torso exists in only two dimensions—think of yourself as side to side, not front to back. Avoid spiraling off your center.

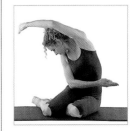

TRANSITION

✳ Turn over onto your stomach for Heel Beats.

HEEL BEATS

The preparation exercise for Heel Beats was V-Pull from the B.E.A.M. Fundamentals (see page 76). As in V-Pull, you will once again engage your Powerhouse to tuck your pelvis while lying facedown on the mat. However, you'll increase the challenge of the V-Pull exercise by adding a scissoring movement in and out with the legs—our Heel Beats!

FIG. 1

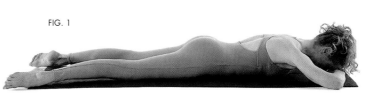

FIG. 1

✳ Lie facedown on the mat, hands stacked under your forehead. Open your legs to the width of your mat, and rotate your heels toward one another. Inhale in home position.

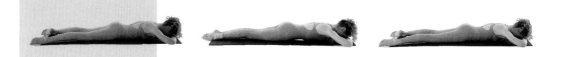

FIG. 2

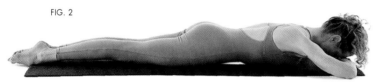

FIG. 2

✳ Exhale completely as you contract up into V-Pull from the B.E.A.M. Fundamentals, creating a tunnel under your navel. Lengthen your legs out of your hips so your feet barely hover off your mat. Begin beating your heels together in time with the "sniff sniff, blow blow" breathing pattern. Perform 40 beats. Rest and repeat up to 3 times.

OPTIONS

✳ If your lower back is tight, place a pillow under your hips (see photo on page 79).

✳ If your neck and shoulders tense easily, place a pillow under your forehead and relax your arms long at your sides.

✳ If you have trouble maintaining your tunnel as you beat your heels together, repeat the V-Pull until you're strong enough to perform both actions simultaneously.

BODY SCAN

✳ Raising your legs too high will cause you to lose your pelvic tuck, placing undue pressure on your lower back.

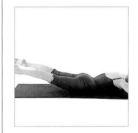

TRANSITION

✳ Press your upper body up and slide your buttocks back to sit on your heels in Rest Position (see page 82) for a moment. Breathe.

SQUAT AND ROLL UP TO STANDING

This exercise begins in a low crouch and ends in your best vertical standing posture. You already practiced the concept of stacking the vertebrae vertically in Spine Stretch (see page 106), but now you'll add the challenge of aligning your feet, knees, and hips as you integrate all the strengthening and stretching from the matwork into an upright stance.

BREATHE

Inhale in the squat position; exhale to roll up to standing.

FIG. 1

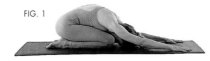

FIG. 1

✳ Begin in Rest Position (see page 82). Focus on deep inhalations to the sides and back of your ribs and full exhalations initiated from your lower abs and pelvic floor muscles. Do at least 3 full breath cycles in Rest.

ENERGIZE

Plant the tripod of both feet firmly on the floor to form a solid foundation. Keep that connection as you unfurl your spine to vertical, reaching the crown of your head toward the ceiling.

FIG. 2

FIG. 2

✳ Arrange your feet hip-width apart, bending each foot at the toes.

ALIGN

Ground the tripod of your feet. Knees track over your toes. Your pelvis should be balanced over (not behind) your feet. Shoulders are directly over your hips.

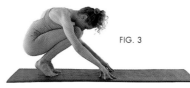

FIG. 3

FIG. 3

✳ Push back to a squatting position, using your fingertips on the mat for balance. Relax your chin down toward your chest.

MOVE

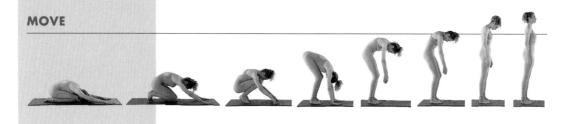

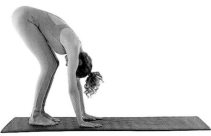

FIG. 4

FIG. 4

* Press your heels into your mat, and hang in a forward fold with relaxed knees. Your kneecaps should track directly over the center of each foot. Relax your upper body and hang like a rag doll. Breathe deeply. On your next inhalation, press your feet firmly into the floor to form a strong foundation.

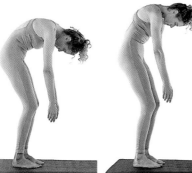
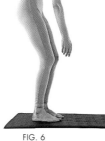

FIG. 5   FIG. 6

FIG. 5

* Exhale to engage your Powerhouse, and slowly roll up to a standing position.

FIG. 6

* Place one vertebra on top of the other.

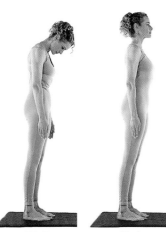

FIG. 7   FIG. 8

FIG. 7

* Your chin should be the last thing to unfold off your chest, as you balance your head evenly on top of your spine.

FIG. 8

* Focus your eyes straight ahead. Feel all the muscles you've worked on the floor support you now in your best upright posture. One perfect repetition will suffice.

OPTIONS

* Walk your hands up your shins and thighs as you roll up to standing.

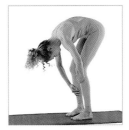

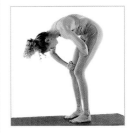

BODY SCAN

* Don't sink when you're in the squatting position, but think of lifting the center of your body the way a cat would when it's getting ready to pounce. This will help you rise out of the squat.

TRANSITION

* Remain standing to stretch and test your balance.

ARM RAISES, SIDE STRETCH, AND RISE

This brief series is your opportunity to integrate all the information your body has learned from the matwork into the upright posture you walk around in. You'll find a standing variation of Arm Raises from the B.E.A.M. Fundamentals, a Side Stretch, and finally a balance test.

BREATHE

For Arm Raises, inhale to raise your arms; exhale to lower. For Side Stretch, inhale in a vertical position; exhale into the stretch. Exhale as you perform the Rise and come onto the balls of your feet.

ENERGIZE

Ground the tripod of each foot firmly on the floor, and visualize a marionette string extending from the crown of your head to the ceiling.

ALIGN

Keep your shoulders vertical over your hips and the points of your triangles overlapped as your arms move.

MOVE

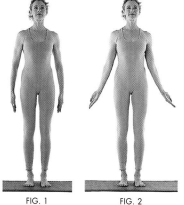

FIG. 1   FIG. 2

FIG. 1

* Stand tall with your arms stretched long at the sides of your body, palms facing in. Your feet should be parallel and hip-width apart. Exhale in home position.

FIG. 2

* Begin inhaling, and turn your palms to face outward.

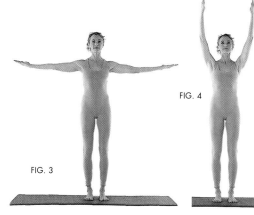

FIG. 3

FIG. 4

FIG. 3

* Continue inhaling as you raise your arms to the side.

FIG. 4

* Complete the inhale as you raise your arms overhead. Drop your shoulder blades down into your back pockets.

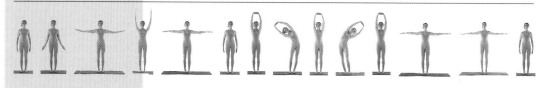

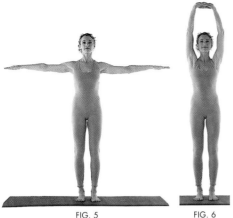

FIG. 5

FIG. 6

FIG. 5

✳ Exhale as you turn your palms down to return home (see Fig. 1). Perform 4 Arm Raises, holding the last one overhead.

FIG. 6

✳ Inhale as you interlace your fingers and turn your palms toward the ceiling. Stretch long out of the sides of your body.

BODY SCAN

✳ In Arm Raises, reach out of your shoulders through your fingertips.

✳ As you lower your arms, feel as though you're pushing through molasses, controlling the movement with your underarm muscles.

✳ In Side Stretch, keep your upper body and hips facing front. Avoid spiraling off your center.

✳ In Rise, feel two-way energy pressing down from your underarms and up through the crown of your head. This will help you maintain balance for a longer period of time.

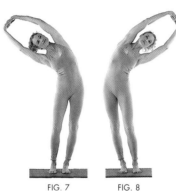

FIG. 7

FIG. 8

FIG. 7

✳ Exhale as you bend your right knee, stretching up and over to the right. Inhale as you return to vertical (see Fig. 6).

FIG. 8

✳ Exhale as you bend your left knee, stretching up and over to the left. Inhale as you return to vertical.

✳ Release your hands and exhale as you press your arms down to shoulder height, palms facing down. Inhale, engaging your Powerhouse and pressing your feet firmly into the floor (see Fig. 5).

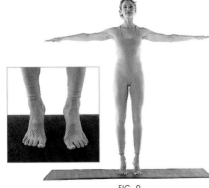

FIG. 9

FIG. 9

✳ Exhale to rise onto the balls of your feet and test your balance. Balance your weight evenly across your forefeet and avoid rolling in or out. Hold your balance for one breath. Then inhale once more, feeling the marionette string continuing to lift you vertically. Exhale to slowly lower your heels back to your mat, arms to your sides, in home position (see Fig. 1).

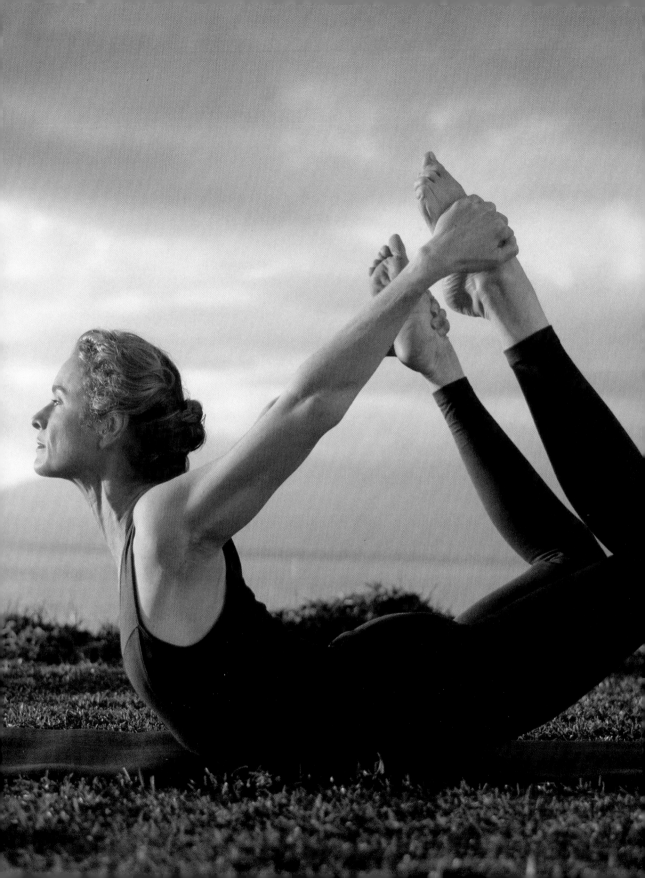

[5]

TAKE 5: AUXILIARY EXERCISES

The auxiliary exercises are four short, simple routines that each take five minutes or less to do. My idea in presenting these routines at the end of this book is to encourage you to integrate your Pilates practice into your everyday life in small, digestible pieces. I know you won't always have time for an hour or even a half-hour workout. But everyone can take a five-minute break now and then. In fact, you may find one of these routines is more restorative than a cup of coffee when you hit an energy slump in your day.

These auxiliary routines will keep the B.E.A.M. Fundamentals and Pilates principles firmly entrenched in your mind and body, ensuring that you walk taller and feel and look better in between your longer mat workout sessions. You don't need special clothing, props, or a lot of time to do these exercises, so there's no excuse not to get to work! Try alternating these routines throughout the week, and you may be surprised at the results. Most important, remember to have some fun!

UPPER BODY CHAIR WORKOUT

If you do a lot of work seated at a desk, this routine is a wonderful way to stretch out your upper body, relieve tension, and reenergize. Try drinking a glass of water and performing the chair routine instead of having a cup of coffee, and notice how much better you feel.

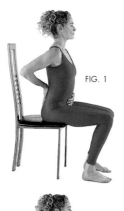

FIG. 1

BREATHING

FIG. 1

❊ Sit on the edge of your chair, back straight and feet hip-width apart. Place one hand on the front of your lower abs and one hand on your lower back. Inhale through your nose.

FIG. 2

❊ Exhale completely through your mouth, contracting your lower abs toward your backbone. Draw your hands closer together, growing taller and thinner. Repeat 5 times.

MOVE

FIG. 2

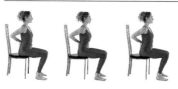

ARM RAISES

FIG. 1

❊ Sit tall with your arms stretched long at the sides of your body, palms facing in.

FIG. 2

❊ Inhale, turn your palms upward, and raise your arms overhead. Keep your shoulders down! Exhale, and return to home position. Repeat 10 times, holding the last Arm Raise overhead.

MOVE

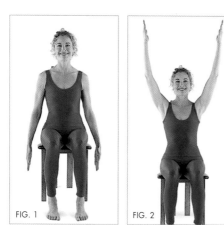

FIG. 1   FIG. 2

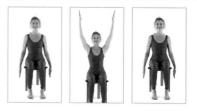

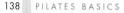

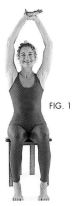

FIG. 1

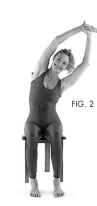

FIG. 2

SIDE STRETCH

FIG. 1

✳ Holding the inhalation from the last Arm Raise, grasp your right wrist with your left hand.

FIG. 2

✳ Exhale to stretch left, keeping your right buttock rooted to the chair. Inhale to back off the stretch just slightly. Exhale to deepen it. Repeat.

FIG. 3

✳ Inhale to return to the starting position and change hands.

FIG. 4

✳ Exhale to repeat the stretch to the other side. Inhale to back off the stretch slightly. Exhale to deepen it. Repeat. Inhale to return to home position, and exhale to bring your arms down to your sides.

MOVE

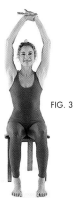

FIG. 3

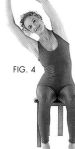

FIG. 4

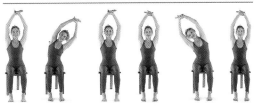

SHRUGS

FIG. 1

✳ Make fists with your hands at your sides.

FIG. 2

✳ Inhale to shrug your shoulders up by your ears, and hold your shoulders very tight and tense. Exhale to drop your shoulders, releasing the tension and returning to home position. Perform 3 repetitions.

MOVE

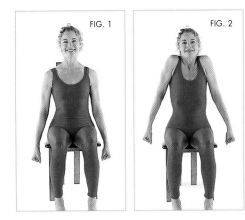

FIG. 1

FIG. 2

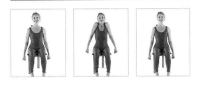

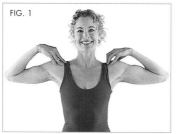

FIG. 1

SHOULDER ROLLS

FIG. 1

✳ Bring your fingertips to the tops of your shoulders, elbows out to your sides.

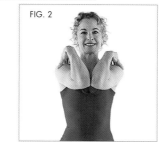

FIG. 2

FIG. 2

✳ Begin inhaling as you touch your elbows in front of your chest.

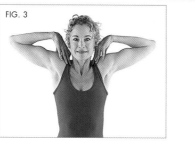

FIG. 3

FIG. 3

✳ Continue inhaling as you raise your shoulders and widen your elbows up and out to your sides.

FIG. 4

FIG. 4

✳ Exhale as you drop your shoulders and circle your elbows around behind you and down toward your waistline. Inhale to touch your elbows in front as you repeat. Perform 4 circles in each direction.

MOVE

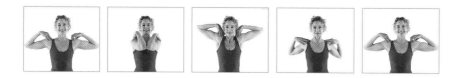

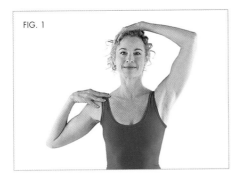

FIG. 1

NECK STRETCHES

FIG. 1

✳ Place your right hand on your right shoulder and your left hand on top of your head. Inhale.

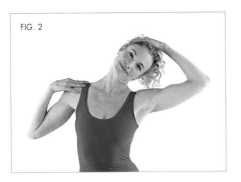

FIG. 2

FIG. 2

✳ Exhale to drop your left ear toward your left shoulder. Do not tip your body—anchor your right shoulder down with your fingertips and focus on the stretch in your neck. Inhale to back off the stretch slightly, exhale to deepen it, and repeat. Inhale to return to home position, and shift your left hand to cradle your head with your fingertips pointing toward the back of your head.

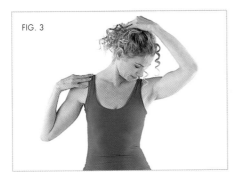

FIG. 3

FIG. 3

✳ Exhale to drop your chin diagonally toward your armpit. Inhale to back off the stretch, exhale to deepen it, and repeat. Inhale to return to home position, change hands, and do both stretches to the other side.

MOVE

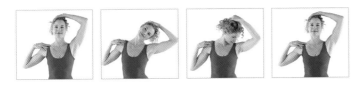

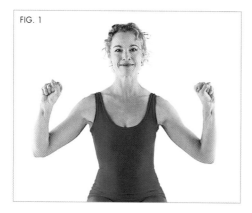

FIG. 1

HAND STRETCHES

FIG. 1

＊Make tight fists.

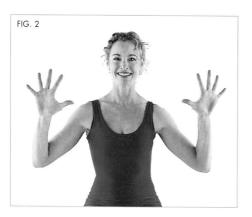

FIG. 2

FIG. 2

＊Stretch your fingers and hands open as wide as possible. Repeat 5 times.

MOVE

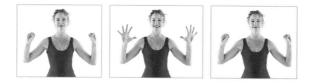

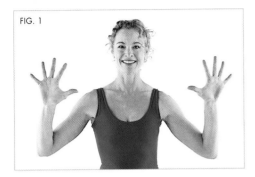

FIG. 1

WRIST CIRCLES

FIG. 1

✳ Begin with your hands at shoulder height, palms facing forward. Keep your fingers open as wide as possible to receive the maximum stretch.

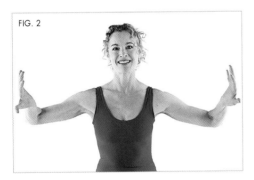

FIG. 2

FIG. 2

✳ Start rotating your hands around to the outside.

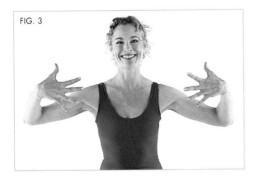

FIG. 3

FIG. 3

✳ Continue rotating down through, palms back toward you, and end up with palms facing out. Rotate the palms of your hands around 4 times in each direction.

MOVE

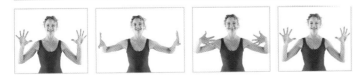

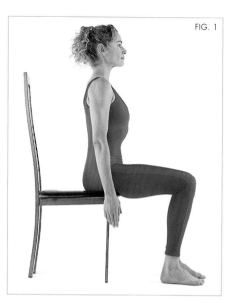

FIG. 1

TWIST

FIG. 1

✳ Keep your hips facing front and your feet planted firmly on the floor.

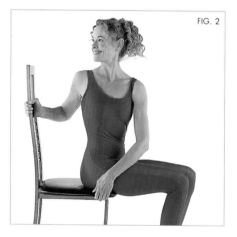

FIG. 2

FIG. 2

✳ Inhale to rotate your torso right. Grasp the back of the chair with your right hand, the front with your left. Exhale to deepen the rotation. Inhale to back off slightly; exhale to deepen. Repeat, and then rotate back to home position. Repeat the Twist in the opposite direction.

MOVE

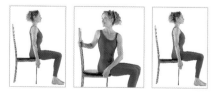

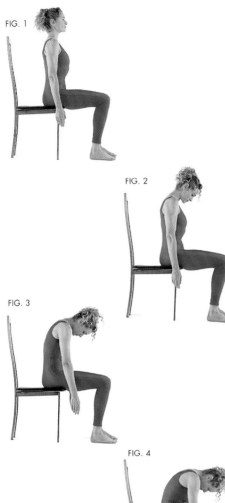

FIG. 1

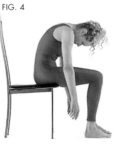

FIG. 2

FIG. 3

FIG. 4

SPINE STRETCH

FIG. 1

✳ Sit tall at the edge of your chair, eyes leveled straight ahead. Keep your hips facing front and your feet planted firmly on the floor, hip-width apart. Inhale.

FIG. 2

✳ Begin to exhale, dropping your chin toward your chest.

FIG. 3

✳ Continue to exhale, dropping your shoulders forward and keeping your arms relaxed and hanging freely.

FIG. 4

✳ Complete the exhalation, rolling further down. Keep your abs pulled up and in at all times! Inhale to restack your vertebrae in home position. Repeat 5 times.

MOVE

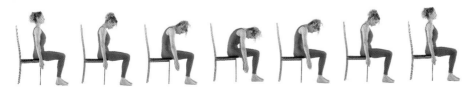

LOWER BODY CHAIR WORKOUT

Chair Squats strengthen your legs and Powerhouse. They include a stretch for your quadriceps, the muscles on the fronts of your thighs.

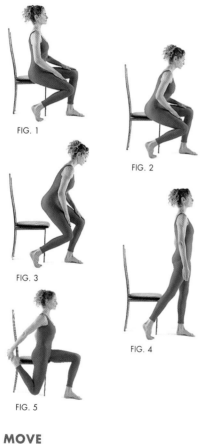

FIG. 1

FIG. 2

FIG. 3

FIG. 4

FIG. 5

CHAIR SQUATS

FIG. 1

✳ Sit on the right side of a chair with your right buttock hanging off the seat. Place your left foot flat on the floor in front and your right foot "on the walk" to the right side.

FIG. 2

✳ Inhale, maintaining a neutral spine, and tip your torso forward from your hips.

FIG. 3

✳ Exhale to lift off your seat. Push with your legs to lift your body, and maintain good alignment.

FIG. 4

✳ Rise all the way up to vertical by the end of your exhalation. Inhale to lower yourself slowly back to the chair. Repeat up to 10 times, and then change sides.

FIG. 5

✳ To stretch the front of your right thigh, bend your knee and grasp your foot. Inhale, and as you exhale, draw your abs up and in as you straighten your knee toward the floor. Caution: Avoid overarching your lower back.

MOVE

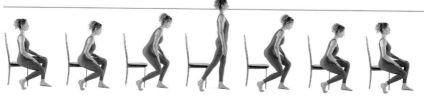

WALL WORKOUT

These exercises use a wall as a prop. Engage your abdominals to press your lower back into the wall, and lengthen your entire spine from top to bottom. Focus on keeping energy in your Powerhouse throughout, and take care not to let excess tension creep upward to your head, neck, and shoulders.

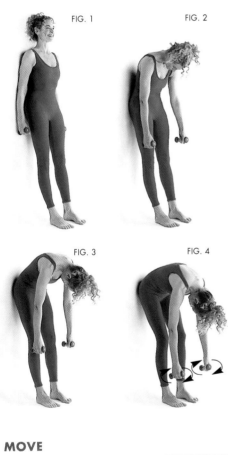

FIG. 1   FIG. 2

FIG. 3   FIG. 4

PEELING OFF THE WALL

FIG. 1

✳ Lean against a wall with your feet hip-width apart. Walk your feet far enough away to flatten your lower back against the wall. Relax your arms at your sides. (Optionally, you can hold 1- or 2-pound hand weights.) Inhale in this position.

FIG. 2

✳ Begin to exhale, dropping your chin toward your chest.

FIG. 3

✳ Peel the backs of your shoulders away from the wall, continuing to exhale.

FIG. 4

✳ Finish exhaling as the backs of your ribs peel away from the wall. Keep your lower abs pulled up and in to support your back, and stretch your spine. Inhale to return to home position, stacking your vertebrae one at a time back against the wall. Keep your shoulders relaxed at all times and your arms hanging limply down from your torso. Repeat 3 times. Hold the last peel away, and perform 5 small arm circles in each direction. Return to home position.

MOVE

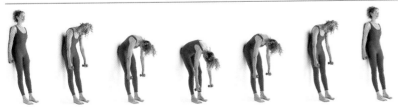

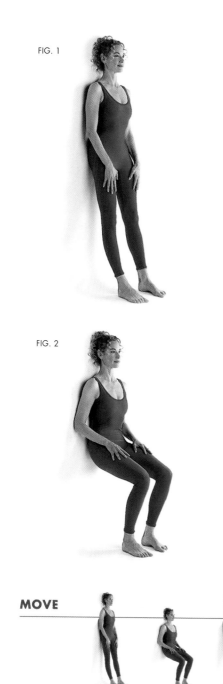

FIG. 1

FIG. 2

WALL SLIDE

FIG. 1

✳ Stand tall while leaning against a wall, as in Peeling Off the Wall (see page 147).

FIG. 2

✳ Inhale and bend your knees to slide down the wall into a squat. Maintain correct alignment of your knees over the center of each foot. Exhale, holding the position and drawing your lower abs flat against the wall. Inhale, holding the position once more. Exhale, engage your Powerhouse, and press your feet firmly into the floor to slide slowly back up the wall. Repeat up to 10 times. As you grow stronger, increase the amount of time you hold the squat. Keep track of your progress by counting your breaths.

MOVE

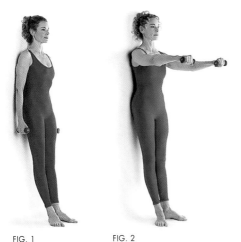

FIG. 1   FIG. 2

ARM CIRCLES

FIG. 1

✳ Stand tall, leaning against the wall in Pilates Stance, arms relaxed at your sides. Optionally, you can hold 1- or 2-pound hand weights. Exhale in home position.

FIG. 2

✳ Inhale as you raise your arms forward to shoulder height.

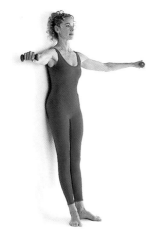

FIG. 3

FIG. 3

✳ Holding the inhalation, open your arms diagonally in front of you. Caution: Don't open too far to the sides—keep your hands in your peripheral vision. Exhale to return to home position. Perform 4 circles, and then reverse direction to perform 4 more.

MOVE

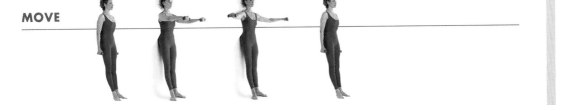

5-MINUTE TUMMY TUCK

The Tummy Tuck is a fast-moving, quick-and-dirty ab routine that will help to flatten your stomach. If you're feeling sleepy but can't take a nap (like when you're at work), try doing the Breath of Fire exercise on its own, and feel your energy soar!

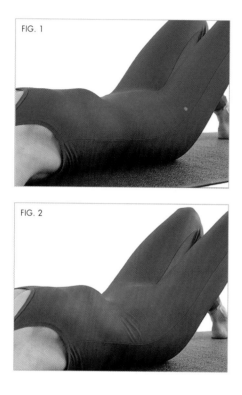

FIG. 1

FIG. 2

BELLY BLASTER

FIG. 1

✳ Lie on your back on a soft rug or mat with your knees bent and feet hip-width apart. Interlace your hands behind the base of your skull, and let your elbows relax down. Inhale, visualizing a long spine from head to tailbone.

FIG. 2

✳ Exhale and scoop your lower abs to press the small of your back into the floor. Keep your lower back and buttocks muscles relaxed throughout, concentrating on flattening your tummy. Inhale, holding the scoop; then exhale, deepening the abdominal contraction. Inhale as you gently release to home position. On the next exhalation, begin the scoop again. Build up to 10 repetitions.

MOVE

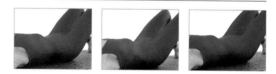

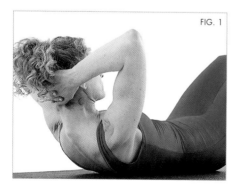

FIG. 1

AB BLASTER

FIG. 1

✳ Begin in the same home position as the Belly Blaster (above). As you exhale, engage your rib cage abdominals and curl your upper body off the floor. Keep your neck graceful and long. Don't pooch your lower abs! Inhale, holding the curl, and then exhale, deepening the contraction in your abs. Inhale as you roll down to a relaxed position. On the next exhalation, begin the curl again. Build up to 10 repetitions.

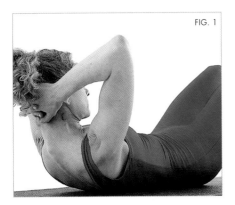
FIG. 1

DOUBLE WHAMMY

FIG. 1

✳ The Double Whammy combines the Belly Blaster and the Ab Blaster. Begin in the same home position, inhale, and then exhale as you perform both movements simultaneously. Inhale to hold the position, and then exhale to deepen the lower ab scoop and the rib cage ab curl. Relax down as you exhale. Keep your lower back and buttocks muscles relaxed throughout, concentrating on flattening your tummy. Build up to 10 repetitions.

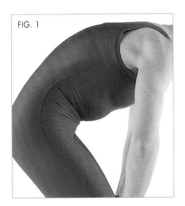
FIG. 1

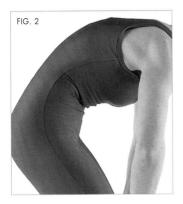
FIG. 2

BREATH OF FIRE

FIG. 1

✳ Stand with your feet parallel to each other and positioned directly under your hip joints. Bend your knees and round your back, resting your palms on the tops of your thighs with your elbows out. Inhale.

FIG. 2

✳ Exhale quickly and percussively through your mouth, drawing your lower belly sharply up into your spine. Perform 10 brisk contractions of your abs. Then inhale to roll up to standing, and relax. Roll back down and repeat the 10 quick exhalations and ab contractions. Build up to 5 sets of 10.

MOVE

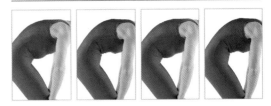

GLOSSARY

Body-mind connection. The state of focusing the mind on the body's movements. An increased body-mind connection will allow clean, centered movement free from strain.

Chin tucked. Tucking the chin elongates the muscles in the back of the neck and can provide a good stretch for those who have a "forward head." However, avoid the tucked chin position when performing Breathing 100s (see page 94) or any other exercise that calls for rolling your upper body up off the floor.

Foot "on the walk." A position where the full weight of the foot is balanced on the forefoot only—the heel is lifted off the floor.

Headlights. Imaginary headlights that shine out from the front of your pelvic bones. Visualizing these headlights will help you to tuck and arch your pelvis until you achieve a neutral pelvis position with your headlights shining level straight in front of you.

Hip belt. An imaginary belt slung low across your hips, from one pelvic bone to the other. Visualizing tightening this belt will draw the hipbones closer together as you exhale to engage your transverse abdominals.

Imprinting. The action of isolating each individual vertebra of the spine, either using the breath and/or movement.

Inner eye. An internal sense of body awareness. Use your inner eye to scan your posture and alignment.

Intercostal muscles. The muscles that run diagonally between each rib (also known as rib cage abs). Intercostals help to control the expansion and contraction of your rib cage when you breathe.

Level your eyes. To focus your eyes horizontally straight ahead of you. Leveling your eyes will help maintain proper neck and head placement, as well as enhance your balance.

Marionette string. An image to encourage lengthening throughout your spine. Visualize a string extending from the crown of your head to the ceiling, suspending your entire spine along its length, from head to tailbone.

Navel to spine. The process of drawing your abdominal muscles up and in as you imagine your navel drawing toward your spine. This is an original cue that was used by Joseph Pilates. Performing navel to spine as you exhale will increase stability in your torso and facilitate centered movements that emanate from your Powerhouse.

Neck lengthened. An element of good posture achieved by sending energy out the top of the head. A lengthened neck maintains the natural curve of the neck and counteracts compression of the vertebrae that can occur with slumping.

Neutral pelvis. The pelvis in its most naturally efficient alignment. It's neither tucked under nor arched back; nor is it tilting to one side. In this position, your "headlights" are level (see opposite page).

Neutral spine. A balanced spine that maintains its natural curves. Pilates encourages you to identify and achieve your neutral spine. A misaligned spine causes compensating muscles to work too hard, which can result in undue stress, fatigue, pain, and potential injury.

Parallel stance. When the feet, ankles, knees, and legs are aligned directly under the hip joints, with the toes pointing forward. For most people, the inner borders of the big toes will be 4 to 6 inches apart in parallel stance.

Pelvic floor muscles. The deep internal muscles engaged when halting urination or performing a Kegel exercise.

Pilates stance. A position of slight outward rotation of the thighs, originating from the hip sockets. When you stand in Pilates stance, the heels are pressed together and the toes point outward at 45-degree angles. When you perform the Breathing 100s in Pilates stance, the position is identical, but the feet are pointed.

Pooched abs. Abdominal muscles that are pushed out. Weak abs tend to pooch, which can strain the lower back.

Popping the ribs. Splaying and spreading the ribs. Popping the ribs weakens the torso and can overarch the back, as in military posture (see page 30).

Powerhouse. The girdle of strength in the center of your body, just below your navel. Engaging your Powerhouse involves the lower abs, lower back, pelvic floor, and smile muscles.

Scooping your abs. To draw the deepest layers of the abdominal muscles up and in to stabilize the body and support the back. This action supports powerful movement emanating from the center of the body and helps to flatten your tummy.

Shoulder blades into your back pockets. An image to encourage upper back and shoulder stability. Visualize your shoulder blades moving down your back into the back pockets of your jeans.

Sitting up out of your hips. An image to encourage length in the spine while seated. Initially, you may need to sit on a firm pillow to do this. Sending energy out the top of your head and down through your pelvis will lengthen your spine and prevent slumping. Sit up out of your hips to achieve a neutral spine in the seated position.

Smile muscles. The muscles at the base of your buttocks, where the backs of your thighs insert into your pelvis. They form a smiling U shape under each buttock when engaged.

Sniff sniff, blow blow. A quick percussive breathing pattern used in conjuction with quick, precise movements. Breathe in percussively two times through your nose to inhale, and blow out percussively two times through your mouth to exhale. Don't be afraid to make noise while you breathe!

Triangles. An image to suggest the internal and external oblique abs, which run on opposite diagonals across the front of your torso. Visualize two triangles: The first triangle uses the horizontal line between the hipbones as its base, with the point touching the navel. The second triangle is inverted, with its point also touching the navel, but its base stretches horizontally across the front of the rib cage (see page 38). *Note:* In the video, I refer to triangles as "the vest."

Two-way energy. The element of opposition used in Pilates exercise. Pressing the feet firmly into the floor while extending the crown of the head toward the ceiling is an example of two-way energy. Opposition creates power in the body, which helps you to focus on controlling your movements.

Vertebrae. The 32 to 34 bones that make up the spine. Between the vertebrae are intervertebral discs that add cushioning and elasticity.

Zipper (zipping the lower abs). An image to draw the lower abs up and in. Visualize zipping up a very tight pair of jeans, beginning at the level of your pubic bone.

INDEX

Underscored page references indicate sidebars. **Boldface** references indicate photographs.

Build a strong Pilates practice!

Easy-to-use, introductory programs and accessories to get in shape with Pilates!

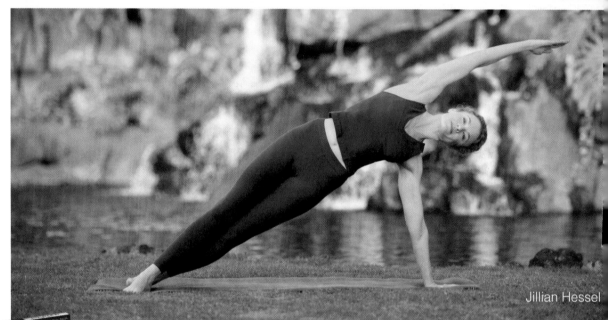

Jillian Hessel

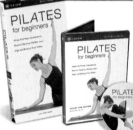

Pilates for Beginners VHS

Master the fundamentals of Pilates and move on to classic Pilates mat work with this comprehensive beginner's program. You learn about posture and breathing and identify the "Powerhouse," build a foundation for Pilates with B.E.A.M. Fundamentals—Breathe, Energize, Align and Move—and move on to a multilevel beginning Pilates mat routine. A great way to build a strong Pilates practice and achieve a functional fitness level that naturally improves everything you do. With Jillian Hessel. *1 hour 15 minutes.*

Pilates for Beginners DVD

The deluxe DVD edition includes pre-Pilates fundamentals and multilevel beginner's Pilates mat workout, separate beginner's modified workout angle, bonus B.E.A.M. Fundamentals tutorial, and an in-depth interview with Jillian Hessel. *2 hours 15 minutes.*

Pilates for Beginners Kit

The complete, easy-to-use introductory kit includes a 45-minute workout video and specially designed Pilates props—natural latex heavy band, durable foam seat riser, and two support cushions for the belly, neck or head—to get started right away.

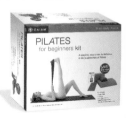

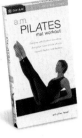

A.M. Pilates Mat Workout VHS

Start your day feeling strong, centered, and energized with this concentrated, thorough program. You begin with a seated warm-up to align your body with the rhythm of your breath, move on to mat exercises to condition the Powerhouse, abs, buttocks and legs, and finish with standing exercises to integrate new learning into your upright body. Continuous movement through each exercise challenges muscles in synergy and builds balance in your whole body. A great way to return your body, mind, and spirit to a natural, integrated state of alignment. With Jillian Hessel. *30 minutes.*

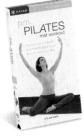

P.M. Pilates Mat Workout VHS

Move from the demands of your day to a relaxing evening and restful night's sleep with this challenging program. You warm up with "The Hundred" to nourish your body with oxygen, work out with vigorous exercises to release accumulated tension, and cool-down by warming and lengthening the spine as you surrender to the wisdom of the body. A great way to bring your day to a joyful end and slip into a peaceful night's sleep… one breath at a time. With Ana Cabán. *30 minutes.*

A.M./P.M. Pilates Mat Workouts DVD

The deluxe DVD edition includes both workouts, bonus Pilates mat workout to energize and de-stress, and in-depth interviews with Jillian Hessel and Ana Cabán. *1 hour 20 minutes.*

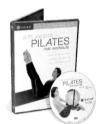

Effective fitness tools to boost your Pilates workouts!

Pilates Mat

Essential to an effective Pilates workout is a mat you can rely on. Thicker than most gym mats, the *Pilates Mat* provides extra cushioning for the back and other sensitive areas of the body while special beveled edges keep it flat on any surface. *Black, ¼"H x 24"W x 68"L.*

Pilates BodyBand™

Maximize your workout with the added resistance, support, and stability of the *Pilates BodyBand*. Three natural latex rubber bands of increasing resistance levels help you intensify your movements and focus your energy on key areas you want to shape and tone. *Purple, green, and blue, 6'L x 5"W.*

Pilates BodyRing™

Enhance your Pilates workout with a lightweight and easy-to-use workout ring! The *Pilates BodyRing* is a flexible metal ring with unique body-gripping pads that adds resistance to your workout so you can target key areas of the body while evenly building strength. *Black, 14" diameter.*

Pilates BodyBall™

Intensify your regular Pilates mat workout with the added challenge of a palm-size weighted ball. The *Pilates BodyBall* is a one-pound, nontoxic ball that helps you sculpt and strengthen muscles, increase flexibility, and improve balance and coordination. *Purple, 1 lb.*

ORDER 800.254.8464 | www.gaiam.com

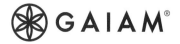

A LIFESTYLE COMPANY
for
HEALTH AND SUSTAINABILITY

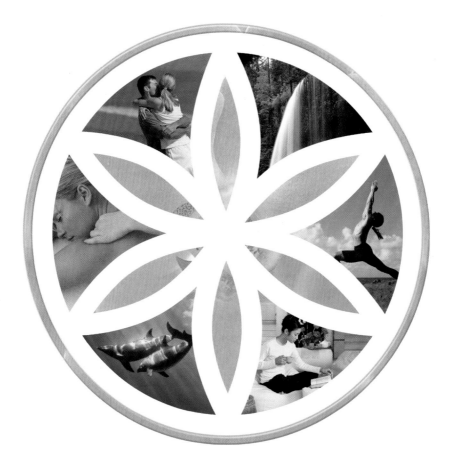

GAIAM®

www.gaiam.com
800.254.8464